100 Questions & Answers

About Managing

The National Lipid Association

Jacksonville, Florida

Editors:

Vera A. Bittner, MD, MSPH

Professor of Medicine
Division of Cardiovascular Disease
University of Alabama at Birmingham
Birmingham, Alabama

Anne C. Goldberg, MD

Associate Professor of Medicine
Division of Endocrinology, Metabolism, and Lipid Research
Washington University School of Medicine
St. Louis, Missouri

Contributors:

Lynn Cofer-Chase, MSN
Laura J. Fox, MD
Matthew K. Ito, PharmD
Penny Kris-Etherton, PhD, RD
Ralph La Forge, MSc
Janet B. Long, MSN

Mary P. McGowan, MD
Peter P. Toth, MD, PhD
James A. Underberg, MD
Wayne S. Warren, MD
Daniel E. Wise, MD
Paul E. Ziajka, MD, PhD

JONES & BARTLETT
LEARNING

World Headquarters

Jones & Bartlett Learning
5 Wall Street
Burlington, MA 01803
978-443-5000
info@jblearning.com
www.jblearning.com

Jones & Bartlett Learning
Canada
6339 Ormindale Way
Mississauga, Ontario L5V 1J2
Canada

Jones & Bartlett Learning
International
Barb House, Barb Mews
London W6 7PA
United Kingdom

Jones & Bartlett Learning books and products are available through most bookstores and online booksellers. To contact Jones & Bartlett Learning directly, call 800-832-0034, fax 978-443-8000, or visit our website, www.jblearning.com.

Substantial discounts on bulk quantities of Jones & Bartlett Learning publications are available to corporations, professional associations, and other qualified organizations. For details and specific discount information, contact the special sales department at Jones & Bartlett Learning via the above contact information or send an email to specialsales@jblearning.com.

The authors, editors, and publisher have made every effort to provide accurate information. However, they are not responsible for errors, omissions, or for any outcomes related to the use of the contents of this book and take no responsibility for the use of the products and procedures described. Treatments and side effects described in this book may not be applicable to all people; likewise, some people may require a dose or experience a side effect that is not described herein. Drugs and medical devices are discussed that may have limited availability controlled by the Food and Drug Administration (FDA) for use only in a research study or clinical trial. Research, clinical practice, and government regulations often change the accepted standard in this field. When consideration is being given to use of any drug in the clinical setting, the healthcare provider or reader is responsible for determining FDA status of the drug, reading the package insert, and reviewing prescribing information for the most up-to-date recommendations on dose, precautions, and contraindications, and determining the appropriate usage for the product. This is especially important in the case of drugs that are new or seldom used.

Production Credits

Executive Publisher: Christopher Davis
Associate Editor: Laura Burns
Production Editor: Daniel Stone
Manufacturing and Inventory Control Supervisor:
  Amy Bacus

Composition: Spoke & Wheel
Printing and Binding: Malloy, Inc.

Cover Credits

Cover Design: Carolyn Downer
Cover Images: Top Left: © Gorilla/ShutterStock, Inc.; Top Right: © Goodluz/ShutterStock, Inc.;
Bottom Left: © Flashon Studio/ShutterStock, Inc.; Bottom Right: © GeoM/ShutterStock, Inc.
Cover Printing: Malloy, Inc.

Library of Congress Cataloging-in-Publication Data
Bittner, Vera A.
  100 questions & answers about managing your cholesterol / Vera A. Bittner, Anne C. Goldberg.
    p. cm.
  Includes bibliographical references and index.
  ISBN 978-0-7637-5679-6
  1. Cholesterol—Popular works. 2. Cholesterol—Miscellanea. I. Goldberg, Anne C. II. Title. III. Title: One hundred questions and answers about managing your cholesterol.
  QP752.C5B58 2012
  613.2'8432—dc23

                              2011010250

6048

Printed in the United States of America
15 14 13 12 11 10 9 8 7 6 5 4 3 2 1

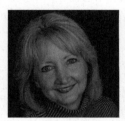

Lynn Cofer-Chase, MSN, is a Clinical Lipid Specialist at Provident Clinical Research and Consulting in Glen Ellyn, Illinois, and a Clinical Instructor at Niehoff School of Nursing, Loyola University of Chicago in Maywood, Illinois. Her nursing career has focused primarily on cardiovascular risk reduction, particularly in the area of cholesterol management and she has been recognized nationally for her work by both the American Heart Association and the National Lipid Association. She worked for many years as the Clinical Director of the Midwest Heart Disease Prevention Center/Lipid Clinic, which received national recognition as a model of excellence by the National Cholesterol Education Program in 2001. She serves on the Board of Directors of the National Lipid Association and the Accreditation Council for Clinical Lipidology.

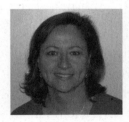

Laura J. Fox, MD, practices at the Cholesterol Treatment Center at Concord Hospital in Concord, New Hampshire. She is certified in both Internal Medicine and Clinical Lipidology. Her areas of interest include overall cardiovascular risk reduction and treatments for the metabolic syndrome. She is an active member of the Northeast Lipid Association.

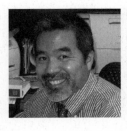

Matthew K. Ito, PharmD, is a Professor of Pharmacy Practice and the Director of the Cardiovascular Pharmacodynamics Laboratory at the Oregon State University/Oregon Health & Science University College of Pharmacy. He has many years of experience managing lipid disorders in high-risk cardiovascular patients and is a certified Clinical Lipid Specialist. He has numerous publications and book chapters related to clinical lipid management and is immediate-past president of the Pacific Lipid Association and current Secretary for the National Lipid Association.

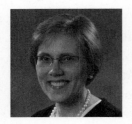

Penny Kris-Etherton, PhD, RD, is Distinguished Professor of Nutrition in the Department of Nutritional Sciences at The Pennsylvania State University, where she has been on the faculty since 1979.

Dr. Kris-Etherton's research has focused on cardiovascular nutrition, specifically on the role of diet on risk factors for cardiovascular disease (CVD) in healthy participants, overweight/obese subjects, as well as subjects at risk for CVD. Dr. Kris-Etherton embraces interdisciplinary research that integrates the expertise of many colleagues.

Dr. Kris-Etherton has served on many national committees that have established dietary guidelines and recommendations. She served on the Second Adult Treatment Panel of the National Cholesterol Education Program, the Dietary Reference Intakes for Macronutrients Committee of the National Academies, the HHS/USDA Dietary Guidelines Advisory Committee 2005, and the Nutrition Committee of the American Heart Association that published diet and lifestyle recommendations. She is a Fellow of the American Heart Association as well as the National Lipid Association, and the recipient of many awards including the Marjorie Hulsizer Copher Award from the American Dietetic Association (2007), the Elaine Monsen Research Award from the American Dietetic Association Foundation (2005), the Lederle Award for Human Nutrition Research awarded by the American Society for Nutritional Sciences (1991), and the Foundation Award for Excellence in Research by the American Dietetic Association (1998). She currently serves as President of the National Lipid Association and Chair of the Medical Nutrition Council of the American Society for Nutrition. Dr. Kris-Etherton has published more than 240 scientific papers and 30 book chapters, and she has co-authored 4 books. Her research program has been funded by NIH, USDA, and the private sector.

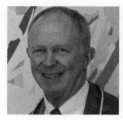

Ralph La Forge, MSc, is a Clinical Lipid Specialist and Diplomate of the Accreditation Council for Clinical Lipidology. He is also a clinical exercise physiologist and former Managing Director of the Duke Lipid Disorder Physician Education Program at Duke University Medical Center, Division of Endocrinology, Metabolism, and Nutrition where he is now consulting faculty. He is also senior faculty for the U.S. Indian Health Service Metabolic Syndrome Clinic Initiative in Santa Fe, New Mexico. He has helped more than 300 medical staff groups throughout North America organize and operate cholesterol disorder, preventive endocrinology, and cardiology programs.

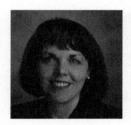

Janet B. Long, MSN, practices as a cardiology nurse practitioner at Rhode Island Cardiology Center where she manages general cardiology patients and also serves as Co-Director of the Cardiovascular Risk Reduction Program. She is the past president of the Preventive Cardiovascular Nurses Association where she continues to serve on the Board of Directors. She also serves on the Board of Directors of the National Lipid Association, the Northeast Lipid Association and the Accreditation Council for Clinical Lipidology. She is a member on the American College of Cardiology (ACC) Nursing Education Committee and the ACC Core Curriculum Education Committee, where she is a faculty member. She is a fellow of the American Heart Association, National Lipid Association, and the Preventive Cardiovascular Nurses Association and a Diplomate of the Council of Clinical Lipidology.

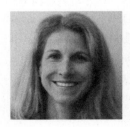

Mary P. McGowan, MD, is the Medical Director of the Cholesterol Treatment Center at Concord Hospital in Concord, New Hampshire and an Assistant Professor of Medicine at the University of Massachusetts Medical Center. Dr. McGowan is President of the Northeast Cholesterol Foundation.

She served on both the NH Expert Panel on Pediatric Obesity and the State of New Hampshire Commission for the Prevention of Childhood Obesity. The commission was asked to advise the state legislature on policy strategies aimed at the prevention of pediatric obesity in the state of New Hampshire. Dr. McGowan also serves on the Board of Directors of the National Lipid Association and Northeast Lipid Association.

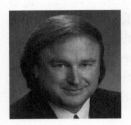

Peter P. Toth, MD, PhD, is a Clinical Associate Professor in the Department of Family and Community Medicine at the University of Illinois College of Medicine and Southern Illinois University School of Medicine. Dr. Toth practices at the Sterling Rock Falls Clinic in Sterling, Illinois, where he is the Director of Preventive Cardiology. He is also the Chief of Medicine and Vice Chief of Cardiovascular Medicine at the CGH Medical Center in Sterling, Illinois. He is a Diplomate of the American Board of Family Practice and the American Board of Clinical Lipidology. He is a fellow of the American Academy of Family Physicians, the International College of Angiology, the American Heart Association (Council on Arteriosclerosis, Thrombosis, and Vascular Biology), the American College of Chest Physicians, the National Lipid Association, and the American College of Cardiology. He is a member of Alpha Omega Alpha, Sigma Xi, and the American Medical Association. Dr. Toth is a member of the American College of Cardiology Foundation Council on Cardiovascular Disease Prevention and the American Heart Association's Council on Lipoproteins, Lipid Metabolism, and Thrombosis.

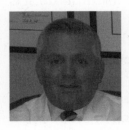

James A. Underberg, MD, is a Clinical Assistant Professor of Medicine in the Division of General Internal Medicine at NYU Medical School and the NYU Center for Cardiovascular Disease Prevention. He is the Director of the Bellevue Hospital Primary Care Lipid Management Clinic.

He is also a member of the executive committee of the Division of General Internal Medicine. His clinical focus is Preventive Cardiovascular Medicine. He is an American Society of Hypertension Certified Specialist in Clinical Hypertension and a Diplomate of the American Board of Clinical Lipidology. Dr. Underberg is the founder and President of the New York Preventive Cardiovascular Society and a founding member of the Board of Directors of the Northeast Chapter of the National Lipid Association. He has been elected a fellow of the American College of Preventive Medicine, the Society of Vascular Medicine, the National Lipid Association, the American College of Physicians, and the American Society of Hypertension.

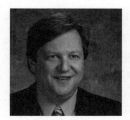

Wayne S. Warren, MD, is a graduate of the Massachusetts Institute of Technology and the Columbia University College of Physicians and Surgeons. He completed his Internal Medicine residency at the University of Massachusetts Medical Center in 1988 and joined Chapel Medical Group in New Haven that same year. He is certified in Internal Medicine and Clinical Lipidology and designated as a Specialist in Clinical Hypertension by the American Society of Hypertension, the only physician in Connecticut with both of those latter two designations. Dr. Warren is an Assistant Clinical Professor at the Yale University School of Medicine and an attending physician at both Yale New Haven Hospital and the Hospital of St. Raphael.

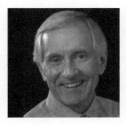

Daniel E. Wise, MD, is certified in Internal Medicine, Cardiovascular Diseases, and Lipidology. Dr. Wise's interest in lipids began with a fellowship at Johns Hopkins and the NIH. He has served as President of the Southeast Lipid Association and on the Board of Directors for the National Lipid Association. His cardiology practice in Charlotte, North Carolina, specializes in preventive cardiovascular medicine.

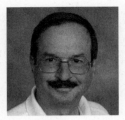 **Paul E. Ziajka, MD, PhD,** is certified by both the American Board of Internal Medicine and the American Board of Clinical Lipidology. Dr. Ziajka entered private practice in Orlando in 1987 and established the Lipid Clinic of Orlando (precursor to the Florida Lipid Institute) the same year. Since 1997 his practice has been limited to the evaluation and treatment of cholesterol and triglyceride disorders. Dr. Ziajka is the founder of Florida Lipid Associates and served as its president for ten years. He is Treasurer for the Southeast Lipid Association and serves on the Board of Directors for the Foundation of the National Lipid Association. He is a fellow in the American College of Physicians and a member of the Preventative Cardiology Nursing Association. Additionally, he is a Clinical Assistant Professor in the Department of Clinical Sciences at Florida State University School of Medicine, Courtesy Clinical Assistant Professor in the Department of Medicine at the University of Florida, and Assistant Professor in the School of Nursing in the College of Health and Public Affairs at the University of Central Florida.

The topic of cholesterol has been of great interest to patients and doctors for over 25 years. Cholesterol is a blood fat, or lipid, that is associated with cardiovascular disease, the leading cause of death for both men and women in the United States and many parts of the world. Cholesterol problems are common and frequently a source of confusion for many people, with conflicting messages from various health agencies and the media about what to do.

Since cholesterol is a topic of intense interest for members of the National Lipid Association (NLA), the NLA leadership decided that a lay audience publication was needed on this subject. The NLA is a non-profit membership association of physicians, nurses, nurse practitioners, physician assistants, pharmacists, exercise physiologists, and dietitians who help manage patients with lipid disorders and cardiovascular disease. The NLA's public health mission is to help reduce deaths related to high cholesterol. We feel that the more informed our patients are, the better they will be able to be our partners in managing their cholesterol levels and cardiovascular risk. Although there are many sources of information related to cholesterol, lipids, and their role in cardiovascular disorders, it is often difficult for patients to find answers to all of their questions. This book is designed to cover most of the questions that patients may have. All of the contributors are health professionals who are members of the NLA.

As in other specialty areas, research into lipid disorders continues at a rapid pace, and new insights into the relationship between lipid disorders and cardiovascular disease may change recommendations for evaluation and treatment in the future. This book should thus be viewed as an introduction to the topic area as the field stands in December 2010, not as a definitive source on which treatment decisions should be based. A listing of web and print sources for further reading is provided at the end of the book. We hope that the book will provide readers with enough background information to be able to discuss their own personal situation with their physicians and jointly with their physician develop a treatment plan tailored to them.

Any proceeds from this publication will benefit the Foundation of the National Lipid Association. The Foundation was created in late 2008 to serve as an education and research organization in the field of cholesterol and lipid disorders, with an emphasis on serving professional, community, and public health interests. The goals of the Foundation are to conduct educational activities, support research, and promote community, and public health activities designed to enhance and promote the key messages surrounding medical efforts to prevent cardiovascular events and death. Readers interested in getting involved in the Foundation can find more detailed information about national and regional initiatives of the Foundation at www.lipidfoundation.org.

Vera A. Bittner, MD, MSPH
Anne C. Goldberg, MD

We would like to acknowledge the contributions of many people who have helped to make this book possible. The list is long and includes National Lipid Association members who wrote questions and answers, the staff of the National Lipid Association and the Foundation of the National Lipid Association, the Boards of Directors of both organizations, and donors to the Foundation. We would like to extend a special thank you to Megan Seery, NLA Publications Manager, for coordinating the editorial process that facilitated this book's completion.

The information included in this book comes from the efforts of many people including research scientists, physicians, nurses, pharmacists, dietitians, and exercise physiologists. It is important to recognize the contributions of patients and their families who have inspired much of this research as well as the people who were participants in the many clinical trials that have advanced knowledge in this field.

PART ONE

The Basics

What is cholesterol?

What causes your blood level
of LDL ("bad") cholesterol to rise?

What should my lipid goals be?

More . . .

Cholesterol

A wax-like, fatty substance that forms part of cell membranes, and that is used in the production of certain vitamins and hormones, such as vitamin D, cortisol, estrogen, and testosterone.

Low-density lipoprotein (LDL) cholesterol

"Bad" cholesterol. A lipoprotein that carries cholesterol to the blood vessels supplying the tissues where it can build up in the artery walls and cause atherosclerosis.

Plaque

Buildup of cholesterol and fatty deposits in the arteries that may gradually narrow the space in the arteries available for the blood to flow to the affected organ.

Atherosclerosis

The process in which excess cholesterol in the body's circulation is deposited into cells in the artery walls, where it gradually forms a fatty deposit called a plaque.

1. What is cholesterol?

Cholesterol is a wax-like, fatty substance that the body needs to perform important functions. It forms part of cell membranes, and it is used in the production of certain vitamins and hormones, such as vitamin D, cortisol, estrogen, and testosterone. Cholesterol is produced in the liver, which can make all the cholesterol that the body needs. It also enters the body from foods of animal origin, including meat (beef, chicken, turkey, pork, lamb, veal) and fish, as well as foods that come from animals, such as milk, cheese, butter, and egg yolks, and products made with these ingredients. Cholesterol is never found in plant foods such as vegetables, grains, or fruits. The cholesterol from the food we eat is absorbed in the intestine and stored in the liver.

2. What is "bad" cholesterol?

"Bad" cholesterol is low-density lipoprotein cholesterol, or **LDL cholesterol**. When you have high levels of LDL cholesterol in your circulation, fatty deposits (**plaque**) may form in the artery walls (a disease process known as **atherosclerosis**). The development of plaque narrows the space available for blood to flow to the heart, which could lead to a heart attack (see Part Two: Cholesterol and Atherosclerosis).

3. What is "good" cholesterol?

"Good" cholesterol is high-density lipoprotein cholesterol, or **HDL cholesterol**. HDL is a much more complex lipoprotein than LDL, but among its many other functions, HDL transports cholesterol from other parts of the body back to the liver (**reverse cholesterol transport**), where it can then be removed from the circulation. If you have a low level of HDL cholesterol, it increases your risk for heart attack and stroke.

4. What are triglycerides?

Triglycerides are fats that are made up of glycerol plus three fatty acids. They are transported throughout the body within lipoprotein particles to serve as a source of fatty acids and energy in various tissues and organs. Excess triglycerides are primarily stored in fat tissue; they can be mobilized when the body needs them as a source of energy.

5. What causes your blood level of LDL ("bad") cholesterol to rise?

All of the following will raise your levels of LDL cholesterol:

- Smoking.
- Eating foods that are high in saturated fat. Such foods include animal products, whole dairy products (for example, whole milk, cream, cheese, butter, ice cream), egg yolks, and some oils, and foods made with these products, including baked goods such as cookies, cakes, pies, and muffins.
- Eating foods containing trans fats. Most trans fats are human-made, not natural products. Trans fats are produced when liquid oils are made into solid fats through a process called hydrogenation. To know whether a product contains trans fat, look for the word "hydrogenated" in the ingredients section of a food label.

High-density lipoprotein (HDL) cholesterol

HDL cholesterol is called the "good" cholesterol because high levels are often associated with a decreased risk of CHD.

Reverse cholesterol transport

An action of HDL involving transfer of cholesterol from cells back to the liver for removal.

Triglycerides

Lipids that are stored in the body in fat cells and used as a source of energy.

- Overweight and obesity. Excess weight can raise LDL cholesterol levels because the extra calories can lead to increased production of cholesterol in the liver and increased storage of fat in the tissues.
- Age. LDL cholesterol levels increase with age in both men and women. After women go through menopause, they sometimes have a significant rise in LDL cholesterol.
- Lack of exercise. A sedentary lifestyle increases the risk of both weight gain and high LDL cholesterol.
- Some diseases and medications. Two common examples of conditions that can cause LDL cholesterol levels to rise are hypothyroidism (underactive thyroid) and nephrotic syndrome, a type of kidney disease.
- Genetic causes.

6. *What causes your blood level of HDL ("good") cholesterol to fall?*

Men typically have lower HDL cholesterol than women. This is due to the different levels of sex hormones, estrogen and testosterone, in men and women. A common cause of low HDL cholesterol is a high level of triglycerides. There is often a "see-saw" effect between high triglycerides and low HDL cholesterol: When one is high, the other is low. The HDL cholesterol can also be low without the triglycerides being elevated, a condition known as **isolated low HDL cholesterol**. Other factors that contribute to low HDL cholesterol include overweight or obesity, sedentary lifestyle, smoking, a very-high-carbohydrate diet (i.e., a diet that is high in processed foods or flour and sugar or foods that break down quickly as sugars in the body), and a diet high in trans fats orhydrogenated fats.

Isolated low HDL cholesterol

The situation in which HDL cholesterol is low, but other lipoproteins are at normal levels.

Diabetes mellitus also contributes to low HDL cholesterol. Some medications, such as beta blockers and anabolic steroids, may lower HDL cholesterol as well. Genetic factors can also make an important contribution to low HDL cholesterol.

7. What causes your blood level of triglycerides to rise?

Triglycerides can be affected by a person's genetic background, his or her lifestyle, and certain diseases and medications. Some people have inherited conditions that are associated with high triglycerides. Triglycerides can increase when a person is overweight or obese, and not physically active. The levels of these fats are also increased with alcohol consumption and in people who eat a diet that is high in refined carbohydrates such as processed foods, products made with flour and sugar, foods high in saturated fat, and sugar-containing beverages.

Some diseases, such as diabetes mellitus, kidney failure, nephrotic syndrome, and hypothyroidism, may contribute to elevated levels of triglycerides. Likewise, some medications can contribute to high triglycerides, such as beta blockers, estrogens, retinoids, thiazide diuretics, antipsychotics, corticosteroids, and protease inhibitors used as treatments for human immunodeficiency virus (HIV) infection.

THE BASICS

8. What is the medical term for having too much of the wrong type(s) of cholesterol?

High cholesterol is often called **hypercholesterolemia** or **hyperlipidemia** (and less often, hyperlipemia or hyperlipoproteinemia). When you have high levels of triglycerides, the condition may be called **hypertriglyceridemia**. The general term used to describe disorders of all **lipid** levels (high LDL cholesterol and triglycerides and low HDL cholesterol) is **dyslipidemia**.

9. Which measurements of cholesterol do I need to find out whether I have hypercholesterolemia or dyslipidemia?

Usually your healthcare provider will ask for the following measurements as part of your **lipid profile**:

- **Total cholesterol** (the measure of LDL cholesterol, HDL cholesterol, and other lipid components)
- LDL cholesterol
- HDL cholesterol
- Triglycerides

In recent years many experts have suggested that non-HDL cholesterol may be a better measure of risk than LDL cholesterol in persons with high triglycerides. **Non-HDL cholesterol** is calculated by subtracting HDL cholesterol from total cholesterol; it includes all forms of cholesterol known to form plaque in the arteries. When your triglycerides are high, your healthcare provider may focus on lowering your non-HDL cholesterol.

10. What should my lipid goals be?

The goals for total cholesterol, LDL ("bad") cholesterol, HDL ("good") cholesterol, and triglycerides are shown in **Table 1**. The goal for non-HDL cholesterol varies based on your cardiovascular risk and is always 30 points higher than the corresponding goal for LDL cholesterol shown in the table.

Total cholesterol

The measure of LDL cholesterol, HDL cholesterol, and other lipid components.

Non-HDL cholesterol

A measurement calculated by subtracting HDL cholesterol from total cholesterol; it includes all forms of cholesterol known to form plaque in the arteries.

THE BASICS

Table 1 Lipid Goals

LDL Cholesterol Level	LDL Cholesterol Category
Less than 70 mg/dL	Optional for very high-risk patient
Less than 100 mg/dL	Optimal
100–129 mg/dL	Near optimal/above optimal
130–159 mg/dL	Borderline high
160–189 mg/dL	High
190 mg/dL and above	Very high
HDL Cholesterol Level	**HDL Cholesterol Category**
Less than 40 mg/dL	Low
40–59 mg/dL	Acceptable, but the higher the better
60 mg/dL and above	High
Total Cholesterol Level	**Total Cholesterol Category**
Less than 200 mg/dL	Desirable
200–239 mg/dL	Borderline high
240 mg/dL and above	High
Triglyceride Level	**Triglyceride Category**
Less than 150 mg/dL	Normal
150–199 mg/dL	Borderline high
200–499 mg/dL	High
500 mg/dL and above	Very high

Adapted from National Heart, Lung, and Blood Institute. *Detection, Evaluation, and Treatment of High Blood Cholesterol in Adults (Adult Treatment Panel III): Final Report*. September 2002: Table II.2-3, page 27 and Table II.3-2, page 32.

11. My HDL ("good") cholesterol is high. Should I still worry about elevations in my LDL ("bad") cholesterol?

Observations of thousands of patients have suggested that high levels of HDL cholesterol have good (protective) effects, and patients with high levels of HDL cholesterol seem to have lower risk for cardiovascular disease. However, your HDL cholesterol level can be increased by other factors, and in some cases a higher level may not always be protective. Therefore, even if your HDL cholesterol is high, your LDL cholesterol level should still be evaluated along with your other **cardiovascular risk factors**. Understanding the cause of HDL cholesterol elevation is key to interpreting its significance.

Cardiovascular risk factor

Anything that increases the chance of an individual developing cardiovascular disease. It may be either modifiable—that is, things or behaviors that a person can change (e.g., smoking)—or nonmodifiable—that is, things that a person cannot change (e.g., age, family history).

12. My HDL ("good") cholesterol level is low. Does this mean I have a problem?

In general, most experts believe that high HDL cholesterol levels are good and protective. Thus, if your level of HDL cholesterol is low, they will discuss this point with you as a health issue. However, as mentioned in Question 11, increased levels of HDL cholesterol are not always protective; likewise, decreased levels of HDL cholesterol do not always indicate a problem. Low HDL cholesterol can occur when you have decreased levels of total cholesterol, as a result of underproduction, decreased absorption, or increased removal of cholesterol. In addition, other causes (for example, other diseases or anabolic steroid use) can lower HDL cholesterol.

Low HDL cholesterol can be associated with increased risk of cardiovascular disease, although this is not always the case. Understanding the cause of low HDL cholesterol is important, as it helps you and your physician understand the significance of this level and decide whether treatments are needed. These steps may be as simple as stopping a causative agent (e.g., quitting smoking or stopping anabolic steroids), or the assessment may reveal a need to treat an underlying medical condition.

THE BASICS

PART TWO

Cholesterol and Atherosclerosis

Why is atherosclerosis dangerous?

How do lipoproteins contribute to
or protect against atherosclerosis?

In the heart, atherosclerosis is called coronary artery disease and may lead to symptoms of chest pain, called angina.

Angina

Deep or poorly localized chest or arm pain that occurs when the heart is not receiving enough oxygen.

Plaque rupture

A situation in which a plaque has part of its covering come off exposing the fatty material underneath. This can lead to a blood clot and blockage of the artery containing the plaque.

Blood clot (thrombus)

Accumulation of material in a blood vessel that either stops bleeding or stops blood flow through the artery or vein.

13. Why is atherosclerosis dangerous?

Atherosclerosis (sometimes also referred to as "hardening of the arteries") is the process in which excess cholesterol in your circulation gets deposited into cells in the artery walls, where it gradually forms a fatty deposit called a plaque. As more and more cholesterol accumulates in the plaque, it may gradually narrow the space in the arteries available for the blood to flow to the affected organ. In the heart, such atherosclerosis is called coronary artery disease and may lead to symptoms of chest pain, called **angina**.

If the plaque continues to grow or if it is located in an area where the blood flow is turbulent, the surface of the plaque covering the fatty contents may become weakened and **rupture**. When this happens, the content of the plaque is exposed to blood and a blood clot may form. Most importantly, a **blood clot** (generally called a **thrombus**) may form. If a clot develops in one of the blood vessels supplying the heart, it can cause a blockage, stopping all blood flow to an area of the heart muscle—a condition called **ischemia**. Such an event may lead to destruction of heart muscle cells, or a heart attack (the medical term is **myocardial infarction**). The result may be that the heart cannot pump blood effectively. Death of heart muscle in a heart attack can also lead to a severe disturbance of the electrical system of the heart or arrhythmia, which can be fatal.

There are other possible outcomes of atherosclerosis. Atherosclerosis in the arteries of your lower legs causes peripheral arterial disease (PAD) and can result in leg pain when you walk (called **claudication**). If left unrecognized and untreated, this condition can be severe enough to eventually lead to gangrene and require amputation. If the arteries supplying the brain become blocked, you can experience transient neurologic symptoms (called a **transient ischemic attack [TIA]**). If not diagnosed and treated, this problem will often result in a **stroke**.

14. How do lipoproteins contribute to or protect against atherosclerosis?

Everyone knows that oil (or fats) and water do not mix. Your body is mostly water. Therefore, for the essential fats, especially cholesterol, to be transported to where they are needed in the body, they must be "packaged" with other substances, called proteins. Such packages combining fats and protein are called **lipoproteins**. The lipoproteins that transport cholesterol and triglycerides inside the body are microscopic particles with one or more proteins (called apolipoproteins) on their surface. Lipoproteins play an essential role in delivering triglycerides to the body's tissues for energy production, in delivering cholesterol to tissues for cell membrane and hormone production, and in removing cholesterol from artery walls to reduce the risk of heart disease and stroke.

The lipoproteins that deposit their cholesterol into cells in the artery wall, which over time lead to atherosclerosis, are primarily low-density lipoprotein (LDL), **very-low-density lipoprotein (VLDL)**, and intermediate-density lipoprotein (IDL). As the cholesterol content of LDL, VLDL, and IDL increases, the risk for heart attack and stroke increases. High-density lipoprotein (HDL) is the lipoprotein that helps to remove cholesterol from peripheral tissue. Thus, as HDL cholesterol increases, the risk for heart attacks and strokes decreases.

Ischemia

A decrease of blood flow to a part of the body due to narrowing or blockage of a blood vessel.

Myocardial infarction

Heart attack or death of heart muscle. In severe cases, myocardial infarction can lead to sudden death.

Claudication

Leg pain caused by peripheral artery disease, in which there is not enough blood flow to an area such as the lower legs.

Transient ischemic attack (TIA)

Transient (or temporary) neurologic symptoms.

Stroke

Also called "brain attack," a stroke is a loss of blood flow to a part of the brain causing death of brain tissue and loss of one or more functions, including weakness, paralysis, loss of sensation or coordination, or the ability to speak or see.

Lipoprotein

Any of a group of protein-covered fat particles that help to transport cholesterol and triglycerides around the body.

Very-low-density lipoprotein (VLDL)

Lipoprotein made in the liver that contains mostly triglycerides and some cholesterol.

Apolipoprotein (apoprotein)

A protein found on the surface of a lipoprotein.

Apolipoprotein A-I (apoA-I)

A protein found on HDL particles.

Apolipoprotein B (apoB)

The apolipoprotein associated with LDL cholesterol and other lipoproteins that are involved with atherosclerosis.

All lipoproteins have one or more unique proteins on their surface, collectively referred to as **apolipoproteins** or **apoproteins**. More than a dozen distinctly different apolipoproteins have been identified, but the two that are most clinically important are apolipoproteins A and B.

Apolipoprotein A (apoA) is associated with HDL, the lipoprotein that provides protection against heart disease and stroke. Although several types of apoA exist, the one that is the primary protein component of HDL has been designated **apolipoprotein A-I (apoA-I)**. ApoA-I is most strongly associated with the removal of cholesterol from the artery wall (that is, reverse cholesterol transport). Most healthcare centers measure HDL cholesterol levels; more recently, however, some experts have suggested that a more accurate risk assessment is provided by assessing apoA-I. As with HDL cholesterol, the higher your level of apoA-I, the lower your risk for heart disease and stroke.

Apolipoprotein B (apoB) is a protein that is found on all of the lipoproteins that are not HDL and is associated with lipoproteins known to promote atherosclerosis. As with apoA-I, some experts suggest that measurement of apoB is more accurate and predictive of health risks than measurement of LDL cholesterol, or perhaps even non-HDL cholesterol. As your apoB level increases, your risk for heart attacks and stroke also rises.

PART THREE

Risk Factors for High Cholesterol and Heart Disease

What is my risk for having heart disease
or a heart attack?

How do risk factors help to decide how to treat
cholesterol? And how aggressively
should we be treating it?

I recognize that I have a high risk for heart disease.
Are my children also at risk?

More . . .

15. What makes my levels of LDL ("bad") cholesterol rise?

Many factors help determine whether your LDL cholesterol level is high or low. The ones discussed here are the most important. Some you can do something about, and some you cannot.

Heredity, age, and gender are conditions that affect your cholesterol levels and that you cannot change. However, it is important to remember that the cholesterol changes associated with these conditions can be treated with medications.

- *Heredity.* Your genes influence your LDL cholesterol level by affecting how rapidly LDL cholesterol is produced and removed from the blood. One specific form of inherited high cholesterol that affects 1 in 500 people is **familial hypercholesterolemia**, which often leads to early heart disease. But even if you do not have a specific genetic form of high LDL cholesterol, genes play a role in influencing your LDL cholesterol level. If a parent or sibling developed heart disease before age 55, then high cholesterol levels—even if they occur just because of your poor diet—place you at a greater than average risk of developing heart disease.

- *Age.* As women and men get older, their blood LDL cholesterol levels rise. Men are at higher risk over age 45 years and women over age 55 years.

- *Gender.* Women's blood levels of LDL cholesterol rise after menopause.

Familial hyper-cholesterolemia

An inherited condition characterized by abnormally high cholesterol levels in the blood. Affected individuals are unable to process LDL cholesterol properly, and they are at increased risk for coronary heart disease.

The following factors are things that you can improve through lifestyle changes:

- *Diet.* Two main nutrients in the foods you eat may increase your LDL cholesterol level: saturated fat (a type of fat found mostly in foods that come from animals) and cholesterol. Eating too much saturated fat and cholesterol is the major reason for the high levels of cholesterol and high rate of heart attacks found among people in the United States.

- *Weight.* Being overweight tends to increase your LDL cholesterol level and lower your HDL cholesterol level.

- *Physical activity/exercise.* Regular physical activity may lower LDL cholesterol and raise HDL cholesterol.

Ravi's comment:

My parents are from India, and despite being vegetarian we have a very high rate of heart disease in our family. My blood pressure and cholesterol numbers are normal and I've been told by several doctors that my risk for heart disease is low. When I told my new doctor about my family history, he ordered a more detailed lipid assessment and it turns out that my Lp(a) [lipoprotein A; discussed in Question 29] is very high. He said this is common in people from the Asian subcontinent and that it explains my family history. Now I'm on a statin and niacin.

16. *What is my risk for having heart disease or a heart attack?*

Risk factors are conditions that increase the likelihood of developing a disease. Some risk factors can be changed, such as smoking and lack of exercise. Others can be treated such as high blood pressure, high cholesterol, and diabetes mellitus. Still others cannot be changed such as age and heredity.

Your risk of having heart disease or a heart attack is determined by your risk factors. Risk factors are conditions that increase the likelihood of developing a disease. Some risk factors can be changed, such as smoking and lack of exercise. Others can be treated, such as high blood pressure, high cholesterol, and diabetes mellitus. Still others cannot be changed, such as age and heredity.

Based on observations of various populations in the United States and other parts of the world, the experts from the National Institutes of Health's (NIH) National Cholesterol Education Program (NCEP) have listed major risk factors for heart attack (and cardiovascular disease). Major risk factors, in addition to high total blood cholesterol, include:

- Cigarette smoking
- Positive family history of premature heart disease (heart attack or sudden death before age 55 in your father or brothers, or before age 65 in your mother or sisters)
- Low HDL cholesterol (less than 40 mg/dL)
- Age (men 45 and older, women 55 and older)
- High blood pressure (higher than 140/90 mm Hg or on medication to lower blood pressure)

If a risk factor can be changed or eliminated, it is called "modifiable." For example, most people can successfully lower their total and LDL cholesterol levels by making changes in their diet, such as eating more water-soluble fiber (in fruits and vegetables) and avoiding saturated and trans fats (fried foods and hard fats like butter and sticks of margarine), and/or by taking medications that have been proven to lower cholesterol levels. Risk factors that cannot be changed, such as your age or family history, are called "nonmodifiable" risk factors.

It is important to know which risk factors you have. The more risk factors you have, the greater your chances are of having a heart attack. Once you know your risk factors, you can focus on those that can be changed and work to lower your risk for heart attack by learning what to do to eliminate those risk factors, or at least reduce them as much as possible. Unfortunately, many people do not know that they have risk factors, and a heart attack may be the first sign that they have a problem. Because heart attacks frequently cause sudden death, knowing your risk factors and making efforts to reduce them can save your life.

17. Some of my close family members have risk factors. What does that mean for me? If I inherit a risk factor, is it treatable?

Fortunately, most risk factors are treatable. Some risk factors are inherited, however. Others are not inherited, but may be linked to behaviors you learned from your family. Risk factors that are passed along in your family may be caused by certain genes, which you may or may not have inherited.

For example, if your father has (or had) a very high level of LDL ("bad") cholesterol and had a heart attack at a young age, his high LDL cholesterol could be caused by a gene that you may also have inherited. In this situation, you should make extra sure to have your LDL cholesterol level checked. To be sure that this test will be accurate, you must have fasted (consumed only water and your medications) for the 9 to 12 hours before having this blood test. If you have inherited a genetic predisposition to high LDL cholesterol, it is important to find out that fact because medications and other treatments can lower LDL cholesterol levels by more than 50%— which means you could lower your risk of heart attack by at least 50% as well.

Another example of a major risk factor that can be passed along genetically in your family is **diabetes mellitus** ("sugar diabetes"). Although you may not have inherited diabetes, you may have inherited some genes that make you more likely to develop diabetes if you allow yourself to become overweight. Excess fat has been linked to a higher risk of developing diabetes, and several studies have shown that in patients who have elevated blood sugar levels (not yet high enough to be called diabetes), weight loss along with exercise can decrease the risk of diabetes.

For example, your mother may have developed diabetes after gaining weight, and you may have inherited genes that make you more likely to get diabetes—but if you keep your weight in the normal range and are active, you can decrease your risk of developing diabetes and, therefore, avoid a major risk factor for heart attack. In individuals with an inherited risk factor, it is particularly important to prevent or vigorously treat other risk factors.

Another major risk factor for heart attack is smoking. Smoking is not inherited, but you are at greater risk if you have learned to smoke in your family or if you are surrounded by people who smoke. If you are a smoker, it is difficult to stop smoking. Nevertheless, many people

Diabetes mellitus

A disorder caused by disturbance of the normal action of insulin (a hormone responsible for lowering blood sugar) and characterized by high blood sugar levels.

have been successful at quitting smoking, and new medications are now available to help you stop smoking. Stopping smoking decreases your risk of having a heart attack.

Finally, high blood pressure (**hypertension**) is a significant risk factor for heart disease and death. The causes of high blood pressure are complex, and some may be inherited. If high blood pressure runs in your family, it is very important that you have your blood pressure checked at least annually to be sure it is in the normal range. Many different treatments are available to control blood pressure, thereby helping to reduce your risk of heart attack and stroke.

Hypertension

High blood pressure. The force of blood through and against the walls of arteries causes blood pressure to rise and fall during the day. If blood pressure remains elevated, it is diagnosed as high blood pressure or hypertension.

18. How do risk factors help to decide how to treat cholesterol? And how aggressively should we be treating it?

Decades of research have taught us that the more risk factors you have, the more likely it is that you will develop heart disease leading to a heart attack or stroke. Some of these risk factors can be modified or eliminated (for example, smoking, or even high blood pressure and diabetes), whereas other risk factors cannot be changed (such as age and a strong family history of premature heart disease). But even if you have many of these risk factors and are at high or very high risk of heart attack because of them, a large number of clinical studies conducted over the past 20 years have shown that lowering LDL cholesterol levels greatly reduces the risk of future heart attack, death rates from coronary heart disease, and the need for heart procedures such as angioplasty, stents, and coronary artery bypass surgery.

It is often difficult to control risk factors such as blood pressure, weight, diabetes, and smoking habits. Aggressively lowering cholesterol levels in people who have these risk factors helps lower their overall risk of cardiovascular disease, even if other risk factors are not changed. For this reason, and because cholesterol levels can be safely and very effectively lowered with diet and medication, the NCEP guidelines recommend more aggressive cholesterol-lowering targets for people who have multiple risk factors.

Although more recent guidelines suggest that LDL cholesterol levels should ideally be less than 100 mg/dL in all adults, the NCEP guidelines specifically recommend that LDL cholesterol-lowering treatment should begin if LDL cholesterol is 160 mg/dL or more in adults who have either no risk factors or only one. For adults with two or more risk factors, the LDL cholesterol treatment target is 130 mg/dL or less. For adults who have been diagnosed with coronary heart disease (or conditions with an equal risk, such as diabetes mellitus), the treatment target is 100 mg/dL or less. For adults at highest risk—that is, those with coronary heart disease and additional risk factors—doctors are encouraged to consider using therapy to help them reach LDL cholesterol levels of 70 mg/dL or less.

Are these very low LDL cholesterol levels safe and healthy? In response to this question, the experts often reply that because our LDL cholesterol levels are approximately 30 mg/dL when we are born, targeting LDL cholesterol to be less than 70 mg/dL should be an entirely safe and healthy goal. There have been no signs in any of the large clinical trials of cholesterol therapy so far to suggest that this supposition is not true.

19. I recognize that I have a high risk for heart disease. Are my children also at risk?

If you know that you are at high risk of developing heart disease and its negative health outcomes (for the reasons discussed in previous questions), then you should also know that your children are probably at high risk for heart disease. Just as is the case for you, some of the risk factors your children face are modifiable, and some are not. Risk factors such as certain cholesterol disorders can be inherited. Thus, if you have one of these conditions, then your child is potentially at a higher risk as well. For children whose parents have high cholesterol levels, physicians recommend they should have their cholesterol levels checked starting at age 2 to see if high cholesterol has been inherited.

Other risk factors, such as smoking and poor diet, are not inherited but can be learned. In this way, you may pass your risk factors on to your children. It has also been found that children who are breathing secondhand smoke from smokers around them are at increased risk for heart attack—a factor that you should note if you are smoking in the presence of a child. Likewise, if you are eating a high-fat, low-fiber, high-sugar diet, this intake has added to your risk, and serving these types of food to your children can increase their risk as well.

20. What are genetic causes of lipid disorders?

A number of genetic lipid disorders, called dyslipidemias or hyperlipidemias, have been identified. Working out how genes are involved in human diseases is an area of active research.

One of the important genetic cholesterol-related disorders is familial hypercholesterolemia. It is usually inherited as a dominant trait—that is, this condition can be inherited from one parent. It occurs in approximately 1 in 500 people and is associated with high LDL cholesterol levels that are usually more than twice the normal level. Early heart disease, with men showing symptoms of heart disease as early as their 30s and women in their 40s, can be seen in many families with familial hypercholesterolemia. If both parents have familial hypercholesterolemia, each of their children has a 1 in 4 chance of having two abnormal genes; if both are inherited, the child will develop extremely high cholesterol levels and very early heart disease. Familial hypercholesterolemia is treated with a combination of diet and medications. Some patients may require a procedure called LDL apheresis, which involves removing blood through a vein, filtering it to remove LDL, and then returning it to the body by another vein. This procedure, which requires approximately 2 hours and is done every 1 or 2 weeks, can be performed in about 50 centers around the United States.

Other inherited problems can cause increased levels of both cholesterol and triglycerides, cholesterol alone, or triglycerides alone. Low HDL cholesterol can be part of several genetic disorders or occur by itself (isolated low HDL). High levels of lipoprotein(a) [Lp(a); see Question 29], another risk factor for heart disease, are also inherited. In addition, some individuals inherit conditions characterized by low levels of LDL cholesterol. Such persons have a lower risk of developing heart disease.

21. I have heard about "the metabolic syndrome." Is it something like having high cholesterol?

The term **the metabolic syndrome** refers to a "cluster" of risk factors that was devised to raise healthcare providers' awareness of risk factors for heart disease beyond high LDL cholesterol levels. More than a decade ago, researchers identified a subset of patients whose LDL cholesterol was "normal" but who were at risk for heart disease and heart attacks because they also had low HDL ("good") cholesterol and high triglycerides, with or without high blood pressure and with or without elevated blood sugar (a sign of **insulin** resistance and/or diabetes). Needless to say, when you are tracking so many factors in so many patients, the degree of variation will be large. Thus the precise definition of the metabolic syndrome—that is, the definition of exactly which levels of HDL cholesterol, triglycerides, blood pressure, and blood sugar qualify for this condition—has proved to be difficult to specify.

22. What is the definition of the metabolic syndrome?

According to the National Cholesterol Education Program (NCEP) and the American Heart Association (AHA), the metabolic syndrome is diagnosed when a person has three of the following five cardiovascular risk factors (note that "abnormal" is defined differently for men and women for two of the risk factors):

The metabolic syndrome

A syndrome consisting of three or more risk factors that increase the likelihood of developing heart disease: abdominal obesity (waist circumference) greater than 40 inches for men or greater than 35 inches for women; triglycerides greater than 150 mg/dL; HDL cholesterol less than 40 mg/dL in men and less than 50 mg/dL in women; blood pressure greater than 130/85 mm Hg; fasting glucose greater than 100 mg/dL; or taking medications for any of these conditions. Weight loss can improve all of these risk factors.

Insulin

A hormone responsible for lowering blood sugar.

- An increased waist circumference (more than 35 inches for women, more than 40 inches for men)
- Elevated blood pressure (135/85 mm Hg or higher, or taking medications for high blood pressure)
- Elevated fasting blood sugar (100 mg/dL or greater)
- Elevated triglycerides (150 mg/dL or greater)
- Low HDL cholesterol (less than 50 mg/dL for women, less than 40 mg/dL for men)

23. How common is the metabolic syndrome in the United States?

Even though there is some disagreement among experts about which measurements should be used to define the metabolic syndrome, there is no question that this condition is common. In the United States, it is estimated that 34% of adults (about 1 in 3) have the metabolic syndrome. The rates are higher among men (35%) than among women (33%) and increase with age (among persons aged 60 and older, more than 50% of Americans have the metabolic syndrome). Among men, the metabolic syndrome is more common among non-Hispanic whites (37%) than among either Mexican Americans (33%) or non-Hispanic blacks (25%). Among women, Mexican Americans have the highest rate of this syndrome (41%), followed by non-Hispanic blacks (39%) and non-Hispanic whites (32%).

More worrying, the metabolic syndrome is also increasingly seen in children. A 2004 report indicated that 4% of 12- to 19-year-old children had the syndrome. Among children in this age range who were overweight, however, the proportion with the metabolic syndrome increased to 29%.

24. The metabolic syndrome sounds complicated. Is there an easier way to find out whether I have it?

There is another way to understand this risk: your body weight. Because almost all these risk factors increase as your body weight increases above your "ideal" weight, simply accurately understanding what your weight is will give you an important insight into your risk level. Of course, people are different, and it is true that some people are just "bigger" than other people. To make allowance for the fact that a taller person would be naturally expected to be heavier than a shorter person, a calculation that adjusts for this factor has been developed: the **body mass index** (**BMI**). To calculate your BMI in U.S. measurements, you multiply your weight in pounds times 703, then divide by your height, in inches, squared. You can also go to the NIH website and use its online calculator (http://www.nhlbisupport.com/bmi/); this site also interprets the score so that you can determine whether your BMI means that you are at risk because of your weight.

Body mass index (BMI)

A frequently employed index of obesity, expressed as weight in kilograms (kg) divided by the square of height in meters (m^2); BMI = kg/m^2.

Finally, if you are wondering whether you might have the metabolic syndrome, you do not have to go to a doctor and have these scientific measurements taken. In several well-designed studies, it has been shown that a very simple, do-it-at-home measurement is equally predictive of heart disease risk: your waist measurement (the first item in the NCEP/AHA list of risk factors in Question 22). All you have to do is run a flexible tape measure around your waist at the level of your belly button; if your waist is larger than 35 inches (if you are a woman) or 40 inches (if you are a man), then you are at about the same increased risk of heart disease and death as if your doctor tells you that you have the metabolic syndrome. Measuring waist size can be very helpful to track progress while working on diet and exercise—individuals often lose fat around their abdomen more quickly than they lose overall body weight (**Figure 1**).

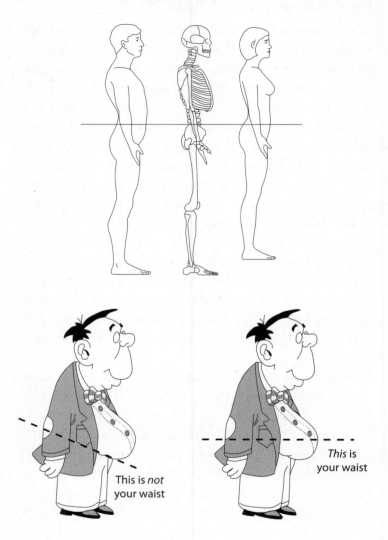

This is *not* your waist

This is your waist

Figure 1 Waist Measurement

25. What should I do if I have the metabolic syndrome?

Regardless of which method has been used to identify that you have the metabolic syndrome, a person with this condition has a greater likelihood of developing diabetes mellitus and cardiovascular disease than individuals who do not have the metabolic syndrome. This is not the same as saying that you "need to lose a little weight." Rather, it means that you have a scientifically documented increased risk of developing illness, or even death, from heart disease. The good news is that the metabolic syndrome is a modifiable risk factor—that is, the risks associated with the metabolic syndrome can be modified with lifestyle measures and with medications. Diet, exercise, and weight loss play an important role; likewise, the blood pressure and lipid abnormalities associated with the metabolic syndrome respond nicely to medical therapy. If you have the metabolic syndrome, you should be concerned and you should do something about it.

PART FOUR

Diagnosis and Testing

When and how often should I have
my cholesterol checked?

Who can evaluate and treat my cholesterol levels?

How can I find a "lipidologist"?

More . . .

26. When and how often should I have my cholesterol checked?

Most people should start getting their cholesterol checked (get a lipid profile) by age 20 years. The children of a parent with a family history of premature heart disease should be checked earlier. For example, if a parent has a heart attack in his 40s, then his children should be evaluated by age 10 years. Children who have diabetes mellitus or who are obese should also have their lipid profile evaluated. Adults who are gaining weight, those who have high blood pressure or diabetes, and anyone diagnosed with atherosclerotic disease in their heart, legs, carotid arteries in the neck, or kidneys should have their lipid profile checked.

If your healthcare provider initiates lifestyle modification to attempt to improve your cholesterol, then your lipid profile should be rechecked 4 to 6 months later. If medication is indicated, then the lipid profile should be rechecked within 6 to 8 weeks. If the dose of medication is increased or if additional medications are added to ongoing therapy, then the lipid profile should be rechecked over the course of 6 to 12 weeks, depending on how treatment was changed. Once a patient is on stable therapy, the lipid profile should be monitored twice annually.

27. If I had my cholesterol levels measured multiple times on the same day, would the numbers be exactly the same?

A lipid profile should be measured in the morning after you have gone without eating anything (fasted) for 12 hours. Lipid profiles after food intake are more variable depending on the type and quantity of food consumed and the time since the food was ingested. This fact makes the interpretation of nonfasting lipid profiles more difficult. Measurement of lipid profiles after meals is sometimes done for research purposes.

28. What is measured when my doctor orders a lipid profile?

A lipid profile consists of total cholesterol, LDL ("bad") cholesterol, HDL ("good") cholesterol, and triglyceride levels. Some laboratories will automatically calculate non-HDL cholesterol levels as well. The laboratory printout may also provide an estimate of your risk of heart disease and list treatment goals.

29. Are there any more advanced tests for lipids?

"Advanced" lipid testing is performed by some lipidologists because the results can provide more information about an individual patient's lipid metabolism than the usual lipid profile. Advanced lipid testing is used to evaluate where specific problems may be occurring in lipid metabolism pathways, such as whether markers of inflammation such as C-reactive protein (CRP) are raised and whether a normal lipid profile is actually masking serious abnormalities in specific lipid fractions such as LDL cholesterol or HDL cholesterol.

A variety of laboratory techniques can be used to determine more specific physical and functional features of the cholesterol fractions in blood. These methods include centrifugation, electrophoresis, and nuclear magnetic resonance. Commercial names for these techniques include the *Berkeley* test, the *VAP* (Vertical Auto Profile) test, and the *NMR Lipoprofile* test, among others. These tests can identify one or several of the following characteristics:

- *LDL particle size.* People have a mix of different-sized LDL particles in their bloodstream. Some studies suggest that "small dense" particles may be associated with a higher cardiovascular risk than larger particles. Although LDL size patterns and the coronary risk associated with them are influenced by genetic factors, this risk can be reduced by treatment.

- *LDL particle number.* This number may be more closely associated with risk of cardiovascular disease than LDL cholesterol level or LDL particle size.

- *Lipoprotein(a).* **Lp(a)** is an LDL particle with an abnormal protein called (a) attached. Elevated Lp(a) levels are associated with a threefold increased risk of heart disease.

- *HDL subclassification.* Like LDL lipoprotein particles, HDL particles come in different sizes, which may be associated with different levels of risk for cardiovascular disease. HDL function is more complicated than LDL function, and is not as well understood, but is the subject of intensive research.

Apolipoprotein A-I. ApoA-I is one of several proteins attached to each HDL particle. The amount of apoA-I may be a better predictor of your level of protection against heart disease risk than HDL cholesterol levels.

Apolipoprotein B. ApoB is attached to LDL particles, with one apoB attached to each LDL lipoprotein particle. As a consequence, measuring ApoB provides a more accurate indication of the number of LDL particles than

Lipoprotein(a) Lp(a)

A lipoprotein particle similar to LDL with an attached protein. Elevated blood plasma levels are positively correlated with coronary heart disease.

a standard LDL cholesterol blood test. Some studies indicate that apoB is a better predictor of risk for coronary heart disease than LDL cholesterol measurement.

Apolipoprotein E. ApoE is an incompletely understood apolipoprotein that exists in both normal and abnormal genetic forms. Measuring this apolipoprotein may identify certain types of inherited lipid abnormalities associated with increased cardiovascular risk.

Current guidelines do not recommend these tests for all individuals. Nevertheless, they can be helpful when evaluating the level of risk in some persons, such as individuals with a strong family history of heart disease at an early age or patients with apparently well-controlled lipid levels but who nevertheless experience a heart attack or other cardiovascular event.

30. Who can evaluate and treat my cholesterol levels?

Most family practice physicians, internists, cardiologists, endocrinologists, and some obstetrician/gynecologists can initiate screening and assessment of your lipid profile. If you have a more complicated set of issues, your primary care physician may decide to refer you to someone in the community who specializes in vascular medicine and the treatment of cholesterol problems—that is, a **lipidologist**. Many physicians are obtaining additional education and training in this area of medicine, and they frequently collaborate with associated healthcare professionals, such as nutritionists, exercise specialists, and psychologists, in a team approach to create the most advantageous prevention program for your particular problems.

Lipidologist

Someone who specializes in the treatment of cholesterol problems.

31. Who decides whether I have dyslipidemia?

The diagnosis of dyslipidemia is based on national standards of what constitutes a normal level for all components of the lipid profile, including LDL ("bad") cholesterol, non-HDL cholesterol, HDL ("good") cholesterol, and triglycerides. Treatment of your lipid disorder is based on your cardiovascular risk (risk of heart attacks, stroke, or death). Your healthcare provider will conduct a risk assessment to determine your specific lipid goals. The higher your level of risk, the lower the levels for LDL and non-HDL cholesterol that your physician will want you to achieve (see Part One: The Basics). The highest-risk patients already have heart disease. Other patients at very high risk for cardiovascular disease include patients with diabetes mellitus, peripheral vascular disease, an abdominal aortic aneurysm, or a history of stroke. The more aggressive the target for lowering LDL and non-HDL cholesterol, the greater the likelihood that lifestyle modifications will have to be augmented with prescription drugs designed to lower your cholesterol level. Sometimes multiple drugs may be required to achieve the lipid goals.

32. How can I find a "lipidologist"?

Most of the assessment and treatment of patients with cholesterol problems can be done by your primary care physician if he or she has enough time to spend with you to assess the overall problem. Some patients have more complicated lipid problems that would benefit from more specialized care, however. In many cities or regions, some physicians may specialize in treating cholesterol problems and be well known for this reason in the healthcare community. If that is not the case for you, other resources are available.

Many of the healthcare providers with a strong interest in prevention of vascular disease and the treatment of cholesterol problems belong to the National Lipid Association (NLA). NLA has members throughout the United States. This organization has been instrumental in the development of training programs that allow physicians to become certified in lipidology (the treatment and evaluation of cholesterol problems). It has also helped develop ancillary programs, which allow other healthcare professional such as pharmacists, dieticians, exercise physiologists, physician assistants, and nurse practitioners to receive advanced training similar to the physician program and become certified as well. Healthcare providers who are members of NLA and especially those who have become certified are excellent resources for further help with your cholesterol problems.

33. Is "high cholesterol" a diagnosis?

Cholesterol is important for normal, healthy body function. It is a building block of cell membranes (cell walls) and is important in the production of many hormones. Elevated cholesterol is not a diagnosis; rather, it is a symptom. When cholesterol is elevated, it is important to understand why it is elevated. Perhaps you are absorbing too much cholesterol from your dietary sources, or you are making too much of it in your liver, or your body is not disposing of cholesterol properly, or a combination of these issues. Understanding the cause of elevated cholesterol is important, because it helps to determine the best way to reduce it. In some cases, elevated total cholesterol levels may not represent an abnormality that requires treatment. Understanding the cause of elevated cholesterol and evaluating the patient in the context of other cardiovascular risk factors helps healthcare providers to make this determination.

DIAGNOSIS AND TESTING

PART FIVE

Ways to Improve Your Cholesterol

What options do I have to improve my cholesterol?

How do we know that lifestyle changes
affect atherosclerosis?

34. What options do I have to improve my cholesterol?

The first step to improve your health is always lifestyle change, including eating an appropriate diet and getting enough exercise. Changes in diet can make a significant difference. Which diet is best for you depends on which cholesterol abnormality you have. Your principal problem may be elevated LDL cholesterol, or it may be low HDL cholesterol and elevated triglycerides, or it may be some combination of these abnormalities. Trying to figure out the best dietary approach can be challenging, but the resources listed at the end of this book can help you with this task. The second part of lifestyle change is increasing physical activity, aiming for 30 minutes of activity on most and preferably all days of the week. For many people, losing weight is part of their lifestyle change. Weight loss also plays a major role in achieving all your cholesterol level goals. Controlling caloric intake and increasing physical activity are both key elements for losing weight. More information about lowering your cholesterol with diet and exercise can be found in the parts of this book that deal with managing your cholesterol with diet (Part Six) and exercise (Part Seven).

You can improve your cholesterol levels by consuming food substances that improve various components of the lipid profile. Consuming adequate amounts of soluble fiber—a type of fiber found in some types of bran, oats (like those used in oatmeal), and dietary fiber supplements (also called bulking agents) like Metamucil or psyllium—can lower total cholesterol and LDL cholesterol by 3% to 5%. Phytosterols (plant sterol and stanol esters), which are found in some margarines, such as Benecol and Promise/Take Control, can lower total cholesterol and LDL cholesterol by 11% to 13% when you consume two to three servings (one tablespoon equals one serving) daily. Deep cold-water fish contain healthy oils known as **omega-3 fatty acids**. Depending on how much is consumed, these specific oils can be very helpful in lowering triglycerides by 15% to 35%. Some nuts (especially walnuts and almonds) have increased amounts of omega-3 fatty acids. Omega-6 fatty acids, which are present in vegetable oils, can be helpful as well.

Some over-the-counter products can lower cholesterol, although you should be aware that claims are made for many products without much scientific evidence to back them up (gugulipid, policosanol, and garlic, to name a few). **Red yeast rice**, however, actually does work to lower total cholesterol and LDL cholesterol. The yeast in this product is the raw ingredient from which one of the **statins** (lovastatin) is derived. Thus consuming red yeast rice is equivalent to taking a very low dose of lovastatin, and may be capable of lowering cholesterol by as much as 20% to 25%. Preparations of red yeast rice vary in how much of these ingredients they contain, however, and some may also include harmful contaminants. It is important that you tell your doctor if you are using such supplements.

Niacin is a B vitamin (B$_3$) that is very effective at lowering triglycerides and raising HDL cholesterol. Niacin is available as a prescription medication but can also be purchased over the counter. Again, not all niacin preparations are equally effective. Use caution in purchasing niacin products. and do not switch brands without discussing such a switch with your doctor.

The FDA does not regulate supplements, which means there is no federal oversight of their quality. It is in your best interest to research any given brand in terms of reliability and quality control. More about dietary supplements can be found in Part Nine: Cholesterol-Lowering Dietary Supplements in this book.

WAYS TO IMPROVE YOUR CHOLESTEROL

Omega-3 fatty acids

Unsaturated fatty acids that are present in marine animal fats and some vegetable oils.

Red yeast rice

A supplement that can lower total cholesterol and LDL cholesterol.

Statin

A general term for an HMG-CoA reductase inhibitor. Statins inhibit the action of the enzyme HMG-CoA reductase, blocking the manufacture of cholesterol in the body, mainly in the liver.

Niacin

A B vitamin (B3) that is very effective at lowering triglycerides and raising HDL cholesterol.

The last step in improving cholesterol levels is the use of prescription medications, which are selected for you by your healthcare provider. Many classes of medications to control cholesterol and triglycerides are available, including statins, fibrates, niacin (nicotinic acid), ezetimibe, bile acid sequestrants, and prescription-quality omega-3 fish oil. Although all of these medications can be used alone, increasingly they are being used in combinations. More about medications can be found in Part Eight: Managing Your Cholesterol with Medications in this book.

35. How do we know that lifestyle changes affect atherosclerosis?

A healthy diet and lifestyle are the cornerstone of our recommendations to prevent and treat cardiovascular disease. People who follow a healthy diet, are physically active, and avoid cigarette smoking live longer and suffer from less cardiovascular disease. Moreover, many clinical studies have shown that when persons at risk of cardiovascular disease switch to a healthy diet and become more physically active, their risk of coronary heart disease events and deaths decreases. In fact, some studies have shown that healthy lifestyle practices can decrease the progression of atherosclerosis, and even reverse it. This effect likely occurs because implementing a healthy diet and a program of regular physical activity improves levels of many major risk factors for cardiovascular disease, such as an elevated cholesterol level and high blood pressure. Hence, a healthy lifestyle is the first-line therapy for decreasing the risk of cardiovascular disease. Importantly, a healthy diet and program of regular physical activity are recommended by many organizations for both preventing and treating cardiovascular disease.

PART SIX

Managing Your Cholesterol by Diet

Can I lower my cholesterol with diet alone?

Which types of fats are there?

How do I know whether I am eating too much?

More . . .

36. Can I lower my cholesterol with diet alone?

Yes. Diet can have a significant cholesterol-lowering effect. You can lower your LDL cholesterol by as much as 10% to 20% simply by changing your diet.

The diet that is recommended for lowering cholesterol is the Therapeutic Lifestyle Changes (TLC) diet developed by the National Cholesterol Education Program (NCEP). The TLC diet includes recommendations for the daily intake of fats, carbohydrates, and proteins as well as fiber-containing products. This regimen basically focuses on the consumption of a balanced diet, emphasizing the difference between "good" (unsaturated) fats, which lower LDL cholesterol, and "bad" (saturated) fats, which raise LDL cholesterol, as well as the difference between "good" (complex) carbohydrates and "bad" carbohydrates (made from simple sugars). Other dietary strategies that can be of benefit include decreasing consumption of trans fats and increasing soy protein intake, especially when the latter replaces food sources of saturated fat.

The reductions in LDL cholesterol that you can achieve through dietary modification are shown in **Table 2**. Diet for cholesterol lowering should be thought of as a lifelong change to a healthy eating pattern, rather than as a short-term effort that will be abandoned after a few weeks.

37. Will different dietary patterns have different effects on my lipid profile?

A number of dietary patterns are known to confer health benefits and protect against cardiovascular disease as well as other chronic diseases. Both the American Heart

Table 2 Approximate and Cumulative Reductions in LDL Cholesterol Achievable by Dietary Modification

Reduction	Dietary Change	LDL Cholesterol
Saturated fat	Less than 7% of calories	8–10%
Dietary cholesterol	Less than 200 mg per day	3–5%
Weight	Lose 10 lbs	5–8%
Viscous (soluble) fiber	5–10 g/day	3–5%
Plant sterols/stanol esters	Add 2 g per day	6–15%
	Cumulative estimate	20–30%

Adapted from Jenkins DJ, Kendall CW, Axelsen M, Augustin LS, Vuksan V. Viscous and nonviscous fibres, nonabsorbable and low glycaemic index carbohydrates, blood lipids and coronary heart disease. *Curr Opin Lipidol.* 2000;11:49–56.

Association and the U.S. Departments of Agriculture and Health and Human Services recommend a similar food-based dietary pattern that emphasizes fruits and vegetables, whole grains, legumes, skim and low-fat dairy products, and lean meats, poultry and fish, as well as fatty fish, and liquid vegetable oils. In recent years, the Mediterranean-style dietary pattern has attracted much attention. This diet typically includes high percentages of plant foods, including fruits and vegetables, breads and grains, beans, nuts, and seeds. Olive oil is the major vegetable oil used. Red meat is consumed sparingly, and fish is a major protein source. The variety of healthy dietary patterns that can be followed offer great flexibility in diet planning, which can greatly improve your ability to stick with a healthy diet.

The nutrient composition of these recommended dietary patterns is similar—that is, they are low in saturated fat, cholesterol, and trans fat, and high in dietary fiber and unsaturated fat, and they should all lower your total cholesterol and LDL cholesterol. If you have high triglyceride levels, you should consume a moderate-fat diet, including healthy fats such as liquid vegetable oils (that is, soybean or corn oil), and not a low-fat diet. Also, you should avoid consuming too many simple sugars because they worsen your high triglyceride levels. Some people are sensitive to alcohol, which can increase triglyceride levels; so they should limit their consumption of alcohol.

Finally, being overweight has detrimental effects on all lipid and lipoprotein level. Just a 10-pound weight loss will lower your total cholesterol, LDL cholesterol, and triglycerides, and increase your HDL cholesterol. Beyond the benefits of losing weight on your lipids, weight loss has many other positive effects, including lowering your blood pressure and blood sugar (glucose) levels. Weight loss also will help your joints, making it easier to move around and be more physically active. As noted earlier, many dietary patterns can be followed for improved health and reduced risk of cardiovascular disease; so enjoy the many benefits of the dietary pattern that is right for you.

38. Which types of fats are there?

Four major dietary fats are part of the food supply: saturated fats, *trans* fats, monounsaturated fats, and polyunsaturated fats. Polyunsaturated fats are further classified into two types: omega-6 fatty acids and omega-3 fatty acids. Saturated and trans fats are solid at room temperature (like a stick of butter), whereas monounsaturated and polyunsaturated fats are liquid at room temperature.

The four major fat classes have different effects on the lipids found in the human bloodstream. Saturated and trans fats are considered "bad" fats, because they raise LDL cholesterol levels in your blood. Unsaturated fats are "better" fats. In fact, polyunsaturated fats (specifically, omega-6 fatty acids) lower LDL cholesterol and are beneficial when consumed in moderation.

Omega-3 fatty acids are found in plant sources (flaxseed and flax oil; walnuts and walnut oil; soybean oil) and in marine sources (fatty fish). Omega-3 fatty acids lower triglyceride levels in your blood. It is important that good fats be eaten in moderation because they are energy dense and contribute calories to the diet. Consuming too many calories causes weight gain, which will have a detrimental effect on LDL cholesterol and triglycerides.

39. Can eating oatmeal lower my cholesterol?

Oatmeal, as well as other food sources of viscous or soluble fiber, lowers cholesterol levels. In the United States, the Food and Drug Administration (FDA) has acknowledged that "soluble fiber from foods such as oat bran, rolled oats or oatmeal, and whole oat flour, as part of a diet low in saturated fat and cholesterol, may reduce the risk of heart disease." This FDA-approved claim, which is permitted to appear on food packaging, is based on 42 clinical studies that, on average, demonstrated cholesterol-lowering effects of oatmeal and oat bran on total cholesterol and LDL cholesterol levels. To carry this claim, oat products must contain at least 0.75 gram of oat fiber (beta-glucan) per serving and be low in total fat, saturated fat, and cholesterol. The 0.75 gram amount represents one-fourth of the 3 grams required to achieve an average 6 mg/dL reduction in total cholesterol. Cooked oatmeal (1.5 cups) or oat bran (1 cup) contains 3 grams of beta-glucan.

Other food sources of soluble fiber may also lower total and LDL cholesterol. These include barley (which provides 0.75 gram of soluble fiber per serving) and food containing psyllium, the husk of the *Plantago ovata* seed (providing 1.7 gram of soluble fiber per serving). It is important to appreciate that other food sources of soluble fiber exist. According to the NCEP, a 5- to 10-gram increase per day in soluble (viscous) fiber intake can be expected to lower LDL cholesterol by 3% to 5%.

40. Does it matter whether I eat fiber? How much should I eat?

Fiber is a very important nutrient. Dietary fiber helps you feel full and is important in promoting healthy colon function. Diets high in fiber also have been linked to reduced risk of diabetes, colon cancer, obesity, and other chronic diseases. The current recommendation is to consume 14 grams of dietary fiber per 1000 calories. Thus, for a 2000-calorie diet, the dietary fiber recommendation would be 28 grams per day. Food sources of dietary fiber include legumes, whole grains, and fruits and vegetables. The amount of fiber is listed on the Nutrition Facts Panel of the packaging for prepared foods, so be sure to read food labels for information about the amount of fiber in a serving of food.

41. Will eating nuts help lower my cholesterol?

Yes. Many studies have shown that nut consumption, in the context of a healthy diet that is calorie controlled, is associated with reduced risk of cardiovascular disease. Persons who consume nuts, including peanuts, four to five times per week are at lower risk for cardiovascular disease.

Many controlled clinical studies have been conducted with different nuts and peanuts, and consistently have shown benefits of nut consumption on major risk factors for cardiovascular disease, including cholesterol levels and blood pressure. Based on this evidence, the *Dietary Guidelines for Americans Advisory Committee Report, 2010* recommends a nutrient-dense diet that includes nuts, as long as increases in nut consumption go along with reduction of calories from other food sources, and reduction of solid fats and added sugars (which provide little nutrient value).

In 2003, the FDA approved the following health claim for nuts: "Scientific evidence suggests but does not prove that eating 1.5 ounces per day of most nuts ... as part of a diet low in saturated fat and cholesterol may reduce the risk of heart disease." The nuts for which this health claim is permitted are almonds, hazelnuts, peanuts, pecans, some pine nuts, pistachio nuts, and walnuts. Other types of nuts are excluded from the health claim because they have more than 4 grams of saturated fat per 50 grams of nuts.

42. How much fish should I be eating and which kinds of fish?

Fatty fish is a rich source of marine-derived omega-3 fatty acids. U.S. dietary guidelines recommend eating at least two servings (4 oz per serving) of fish—preferably oily fish like salmon, herring, or mackerel—per week for prevention of coronary artery disease in adults. For those patients with coronary artery disease, the AHA recommends 1 gram of eicosapentaenoic acid (EPA) and docosahexaenoic acid (DHA) as fish or as a fish oil supplement (see Part Nine: Cholesterol-Lowering Dietary Supplements).

43. Are there any differences between farm-raised and wild-caught fish?

The nutrient composition—especially the fatty acid composition—of fish, both farm raised and wild caught, reflects the diet they consume. Salmon require long-chain omega-3 fatty acids in their diets. Consequently, farm-raised salmon are fed food sources of long chain omega-3 fatty acids. Thus, in terms of long-chain omega-3 fatty acids (EPA and DHA), concentrations in farm-raised and wild-caught salmon are similar. In contrast, farm-raised channel catfish are fed a diet low in long-chain omega-3 fatty acids, and consequently are appreciably lower in these fatty acids compared to wild-caught channel catfish.

44. Is there any danger from environmental contaminants such as mercury in fish?

The best general advice is to enjoy a variety of fish, at least twice per week. To reduce your exposure to other environmental contaminants, you may want to eat smaller fish. Cleaning and cooking fish in a manner that removes fat and organs is an effective way to reduce other contaminants that may be present in fish. Pregnant and nursing women, young children, and nonpregnant women of childbearing age can benefit from eating seafood and can also reduce their exposure to the harmful effects of mercury if they consume no more than 12 oz (two average meals) per week of a variety of most cooked seafood, with the exception of white (albacore) tuna. Young children should be fed smaller portions of fish. All vulnerable groups are advised to avoid consuming certain species known to contain higher levels of mercury, including shark, swordfish, king mackerel, and tile fish.

45. How do I know whether I am eating too much?

The answer to this question is very straightforward: If you are eating too much, you will gain weight. For good health, it is very important to avoid gaining weight. Because it is difficult for many people to lose weight and maintain a reduced body weight, preventing weight gain is recommended. Once you know how many calories you need to maintain your current weight, be careful not to overshoot your daily calorie allowance. Be mindful of portion sizes and calorie-dense foods such as solid fats and added sugars, which add a lot of calories to your daily intake. Instead, fill up on nutrient-dense fruits and vegetables, which are low in calories. Don't forget that juices, soft drinks, creamy coffee drinks, alcohol, and other beverages can contribute many calories to your diet. Make sure that you account for these sources of calories when planning your daily food intake.

If you are overweight (and 67% of Americans are), it is advised that you first put the brakes on gaining additional weight, and then aggressively work toward losing weight. To lose 1 pound per week, consume 500 fewer calories per day. To lose 2 pounds per week, consume 1000 fewer calories per day. Also, start and maintain a program of regular physical activity; it will help you burn calories and ensure that you receive the cardiovascular health benefits of exercise.

46. What role could weight loss play in improving my cholesterol?

Weight loss—even the loss of just a small amount—decreases total cholesterol, LDL cholesterol, and triglycerides. For example, a 10-pound weight loss can result in a 5% to 8% reduction in LDL cholesterol. Weight loss also increases HDL cholesterol.

Having excess body weight around your waist, versus around your hips, increases the risk of cardiovascular disease. Individuals with this body type typically have high triglyceride levels and low HDL cholesterol levels. In addition, they frequently have elevated blood pressure and glucose levels. Not only is the risk of cardiovascular disease increased in these individuals, but they are at higher risk for diabetes as well. Several major clinical trials have shown that weight loss of approximately 7% of total body weight can normalize these risk factors. In the studies, weight loss was achieved the "old-fashioned" way—with diet and physical activity. In other words, participants in the studies reduced their calorie intake and expended more calories via exercise.

47. What is the best diet for weight loss?

There is no single diet that is ideal for weight loss. The important point is to find one that works for you and stick with it.

There is no single diet that is ideal for weight loss. The *Dietary Guidelines for Americans Advisory Committee Report, 2010* noted that high-protein, low-carbohydrate diets may result in faster short-term weight loss, but they are not any better in the long run than other diets. A very large research study found that reduced-calorie diets that vary in their fat, carbohydrate, and protein content have comparable effects on weight loss. Consequently, there is flexibility in designing diets that promote weight loss. The important point is to find one that works for you and stick with it.

It is best not to restrict calories too much or restrict consumption of specific nutrients and foods (that is, you should avoid extremes or fad diets), because continuing with the weight loss diet for a long time is important for success. Thus a balanced diet that has approximately 500 to 1000 *fewer* calories per day (compared to your habitual intake) should result in a 1- to 2-pound weight loss per week. You can achieve a deficit of 500 to 1000 calories per day by reducing your calorie intake by this amount and/or increasing physical activity to help achieve your daily calorie goal.

48. Will I have more success if I join a diet group?

Group-based approaches have been successful for weight loss. Although the details of the programs vary, they tend to incorporate common themes such as education, counseling strategies, behavior change strategies such as goal setting, and self-monitoring. Some group-based programs teach specific skills such as food label reading, grocery shopping, and methods for healthy cooking as well as the use of pedometers, exercise bands or other exercise equipment, and walking groups. Commercial programs that use a group approach and a self-monitoring system to guide food restrictions appear to be more effective than self-help approaches.

PART SEVEN

Managing Your Cholesterol with Physical Activity/Exercise

Which type of physical activity is best for reducing cholesterol and triglycerides?

How much exercise or physical activity should I do to manage my cholesterol?

What is considered moderate versus vigorous physical activity?

More . . .

49. Which type of physical activity is best for reducing cholesterol and triglycerides?

One of the more successful types of exercise being employed for weight control and for individuals with lipid disorders is variable-terrain walking/hiking, where the person walks 2 to 5 miles per day over hilly terrain. The hills add more effort and burn more calories for a given walking distance and can break up the boredom of walking the same flat course.

Almost any form of physical activity will help improve your lipid levels as long as it is of sufficient quantity, which means that you expend enough calories. Most cholesterol disorders respond to the volume or amount of exercise (total caloric cost of activity) rather than specific types of exercise. That said, aerobic activity using large muscle groups—such as walking, running, swimming, cycling, dancing, or hiking—represents perhaps the best form of exercise in the sense that these activities all require significant energy expenditures. One of the more successful types of exercise being employed for weight control and for individuals with lipid disorders is variable-terrain walking/hiking, where the person walks 2 to 5 miles per day over hilly terrain. The hills add more effort and burn more calories for a given walking distance and can break up the boredom of walking the same flat course.

50. How much exercise or physical activity should I do to manage my cholesterol?

The answer to this question depends, to some extent, on which cholesterol lipid measure you are attempting to change. Based on scientific evidence, the American College of Sports Medicine recommends the following regimen:

- Primary activity: Aerobic exercise (for example, walking, jogging, cycling, dancing)
- Intensity: 40% to 70% of aerobic capacity
- Frequency: 5 or more days per week
- Duration: 40 to 60 minutes (but this does not have to be done all at one time)

This amount of physical activity is consistent with recommendations for long-term weight control: 200 to 300 minutes per week of moderate physical activity or at least 2000 kilocalories (kcal; a measure of energy) of exercise per week.

51. Can I reduce all my LDL ("bad") cholesterol and my triglycerides by exercising?

Moderately elevated triglycerides (150 to 200 mg/dL) are perhaps the easiest of the blood lipids to manage with physical activity. Lowering LDL cholesterol is more difficult, usually requiring associated fat weight loss. Raising HDL cholesterol, depending on its initial level, requires at least 1000 kcal of exercise per week (approximately 8 to 10 miles of walking and may increase more when exercise is in the moderate-to-vigorous intensity range). The following are examples of activities that use approximately 1000 kcal of energy, based on a 160-pound person; if you are heavier, the caloric cost is greater:

- 10 miles of walking at 2 miles per hour
- 2.5 to 4 hours of continuous exercise at 55% to 66% of maximum effort level
- Three 45- to 60-minute aerobics classes
- A 3-hour hike over variable terrain with a 10-pound backpack
- 3 hours of cycling at 10 to 12 miles per hour
- 3 sets of singles tennis
- 3 miles of freestyle swimming for women or 2.5 miles of freestyle swimming for men

You do not have to do these activities all at once—you can spread them out over the course of 1 week.

52. What is considered moderate versus vigorous physical activity?

Moderate physical activity is usually the recommended level of activity, at least in the beginning stages of an activity program. Moderate exercise is a level of activity intensity between 40% and 60% of aerobic capacity—in other words, between 40% and 60% of "effort max" (that is, brisk walking). Vigorous exercise is any activity that requires more than 60% of aerobic capacity, such as jogging. This percentage is not to be confused with the percentage of maximum heart rate, which is 10% to 12% higher than your aerobic capacity maximum. Low-intensity exercise is usually defined as physical activity that requires 20% to 40% of aerobic capacity (such as strolling or light housework).

53. Is there a difference in the amount of physical activity required to reduce weight versus the amount to reduce the risk of coronary heart disease?

Generally a larger amount of exercise is required for significant weight loss (2000 kcal per week or more) compared with the amount required to reduce the risk of heart disease, for example (1000 to 1500 kcal per week). It is also true that the more weekly physical activity, the better the effects on both risk reduction and weight loss.

54. Do activities such as yoga, tai chi, and Pilates-type exercise programs reduce the risk of heart disease?

Yoga and tai chi, when properly practiced, can reduce stress and tension; these factors are known to contribute to chronic disease, including cardiovascular disease. For these kinds of programs to contribute to reducing blood lipids, you must follow the same weekly energy expenditure guidelines as for conventional aerobic activities—that is, 1500 to 2000 kcal per week or more. This would require a daily yoga or tai chi practice at a considerable level.

PART EIGHT

Managing Your Cholesterol with Medications

What are statins and how do they work?

I have heard that ezetimibe is an alternative to statins that can lower my cholesterol just as well. What is ezetimibe and how does it work?

What is niacin (nicotinic acid) and how does it work?

More . . .

55. What should I tell my healthcare provider before I start taking medication to improve my cholesterol?

You should be sure to tell your healthcare provider about all other medications and supplements you are taking before starting on any new therapy. If you have severe liver disease, a stomach ulcer, or active bleeding, be sure that your healthcare provider is aware of this fact. If you have diabetes, tell your healthcare provider about any changes in your blood sugar levels.

You should not start taking a medication to improve your cholesterol if you have reason to think that you might be allergic to any of these drugs. Women should be sure to tell their healthcare providers if they are pregnant, or plan to become pregnant during treatment, because some drugs may harm the fetus. Also, if women are breast-feeding, some medications can pass into human milk and may harm a nursing baby.

56. What are statins and how do they work?

Statins are a class of drugs prescribed to lower blood levels of LDL ("bad") cholesterol. They work primarily by inhibiting one of the body's key enzymes—**hydroxymethylglutaryl coenzyme-A reductase** (**HMG-CoA reductase**), which works in the liver to produce cholesterol. Blocking this enzyme causes the liver to have less cholesterol available and leads to the liver removing more cholesterol from the blood. Currently, seven different **HMG-CoA reductase inhibitors** (statins) are available on a prescription basis in the United States (**Table 3**).

Hydroxymethyl-glutaryl coenzyme-A reductase (HMG-CoA reductase)

One of the body's key enzymes, which works in the liver to produce cholesterol.

HMG-CoA reductase inhibitors

Medications that lower the level of LDL cholesterol and are the most commonly used medications to treat high cholesterol levels.

Table 3 Statins Available in the United States

Statin	U.S. Brand Names
Atorvastatin	*Lipitor*
Fluvastatin	*Lescol, Lescol XL*
Lovastatin	*Altocor, Altoprev, Mevacor*
Pitavastatin	*Livalo*
Pravastatin	*Pravachol*
Rosuvastatin	*Crestor*
Simvastatin	*Zocor*

Fixed-dose combination medications that include a statin are *Vytorin* (simvastatin and ezetimibe), *Simcor* (extended-release niacin and simvastatin), *Advicor* (extended-release niacin and lovastatin) and *Caduet* (atorvastatin and amlodipine [a blood pressure medication]).

57. Are all statins the same?

The first statins that were used (for example, lovastatin) were not as powerful in lowering LDL cholesterol as the statins that became available later. For this reason, lower doses of the newer statins may produce the same LDL-lowering effect as higher doses of the earlier statins However, some of the earlier statins are now available as generic drugs, which means that they are produced and sold (under different brand names) by other companies in addition to their original manufacturers. After your healthcare provider has measured your LDL cholesterol levels, he or she will discuss with you how much lower your level needs to be, and this goal will help to determine whether it is better to take a higher dose of one of the older statins or a lower dose of one of the newer statins. This discussion will also allow you and your healthcare provider to take into consideration comparative costs, coverage by health insurance, and availability.

58. Which benefits can I expect from taking a statin?

Statins have been shown to prevent heart attacks, most forms of stroke, and death due to most types of heart disease in adults of all ages, in women and men, in patients with diabetes or high blood pressure, and in people with or without a history of heart disease. The benefits of statins far outweigh any risk of side effects in the vast majority of patients.

Statins have been shown, in many very large and well-known clinical trials, to be among the safest and most effective drugs that your healthcare provider can prescribe for you. For almost all people, therefore, statin medications are safe and well tolerated. Statins have been shown to prevent heart attacks, most forms of stroke, and death due to most types of heart disease in adults of all ages, in women and men, in patients with diabetes or high blood pressure, and in people with or without a history of heart disease. The benefits of statins far outweigh any risk of side effects in the vast majority of patients.

59. What are the main side effects that I should look out for if my healthcare provider prescribes a statin?

Like all medications, statins have been associated with a few major side effects. Probably the two most important are an increase in certain liver enzymes and unusual muscle-related aches and pains. An elevation in liver enzymes occurs in 1% to 2% of patients taking a statin, although generally only in people taking higher doses. It is detected with blood tests and is reversible when the statin dose is lowered or the statin is stopped. Having muscle-related aches, pains, or weakness over and above the ordinary pains associated with getting older and with physical exertion is known as **myopathy**. Myopathy is a broad term that refers to several different clinical situations:

- **Myalgia**: muscle aches or weakness without changes in muscle cells
- **Myositis**: muscle symptoms with an increase in blood tests of muscle enzymes indicating inflammation
- **Rhabdomyolysis**: muscle symptoms associated with severe elevation of muscle enzymes and evidence of kidney failure—this is a medical emergency

The risk of myopathy depends on many factors. Elderly patients and women are at increased risk for this side effect. Conditions such as underlying muscle disease, liver and kidney disease, and an underactive thyroid can contribute to its occurrence as well. Certain medications—most notably, gemfibrozil, cyclosporine, warfarin, calcium-channel blockers, amiodarone, and nefazadone—as well as certain antibiotics and HIV-targeting drugs, when used with statin drugs, can increase the risk of developing myopathy. Recently, genetic factors have also been found to play a role in determining who develops myopathy.

Tony's comment:

After about 1 year of taking simvastatin, I developed fairly severe right shoulder and arm pain. My doctor said he did not think it was due to the cholesterol medication, and he gave me some pain relievers. After a few weeks, it was only slightly better, so I insisted on stopping the medication. This didn't help either, so I went back on the cholesterol medication and saw an orthopedist. After one shoulder injection, I was pain free, and have remained that way ever since.

Myopathy

Any disease of muscles. Symptoms include limb and respiratory weakness. Myopathy can result from endocrine disorders, metabolic disorders, infection, or inflammation of the muscle.

Myalgia

Muscle ache or weakness that occurs without changes in muscle cells.

Myositis

Muscle symptoms with an increase in blood tests of muscle enzymes indicating inflammation.

Rhabdomyolysis

A creatine kinase (CK) level greater than 10,000 IU/L, or myopathy plus end organ damage indicated by a significant elevation of serum creatinine.

60. What should I do if I have elevations of my liver enzymes while I am taking a statin?

If a test shows that your liver enzymes are elevated, your healthcare provider will probably repeat the blood test. Often, the follow-up test is normal even without you making any changes. If liver enzyme abnormalities persist, your healthcare provider will probably either decrease the dose of the stain you are taking or, if possible, switch your prescription to a different statin. Your healthcare provider may also suggest that you take a "drug holiday"—that is, stop taking the statin for a period of time, probably a few weeks. One of these approaches will almost always resolve the problem with the liver enzymes. In extremely rare cases, an elevation of the liver enzymes has been associated with liver damage; this condition will also usually return to normal after use of the statin is discontinued.

61. What should I do if I think I am having muscle pain caused by my statin?

Muscle symptoms should be reported promptly to your healthcare provider. If the symptoms are related to medication, they will generally be present in multiple areas of the body. Pain in a single joint or body part such as an arm or knee is less likely to be due to cholesterol-lowering medication. If your symptoms are consistent with myopathy, your healthcare provider will likely want to order some blood work, including measurement of your creatine kinase level (CK, a muscle function test), tests of thyroid function, and sometimes tests of kidney function. Your physician *may* also stop your medicine, at least temporarily.

If the blood tests are normal and your symptoms do not resolve while you are off treatment, it may be appropriate to restart your cholesterol-lowering medication. In such a case, your muscle symptoms are likely caused by something else, which will need to be investigated. Mild elevations of muscle enzyme are common in everyday life, especially in active individuals. It is not advisable to ask for this test routinely in patients who have no complaints. If symptoms or CK abnormalities resolve after discontinuing the cholesterol-lowering medication, the same medication may be restarted at a lower dose, or a different medication can be used. In as many as 80% of patients, one of these approaches will result in successful resolution without any recurrence of muscle problems.

If you are suffering muscle pains that are truly caused by your statin prescription, then this effect may be due to actual damage brought about by breakdown of muscle tissue. In very rare cases (1 out of 1 million prescriptions), death has occurred due to severe muscle damage and kidney failure. Your healthcare provider will monitor you closely for these side effects, but you should also notify your healthcare provider and/or pharmacist if you experience muscle pain, tenderness, or weakness for which there is no obvious explanation.

62. I love grapefruit juice. My pharmacist said that I should not drink grapefruit juice if I am taking statin medications—is this true?

Grapefruit juice contains a chemical that prevents the body's breakdown of some statin medications, specifically lovastatin (Altocor, Altoprev, Mevacor), simvastatin

(Zocor), and atorvastatin (Lipitor). While this interaction is most pronounced with reconstituted frozen concentrate, drinking freshly squeezed grapefruit juice or eating the fruit itself is also likely to have a similar but milder effect.

As yet, researchers have not determined a specific amount of grapefruit juice that might be safe to consume when patients are on these particular statins. High levels of the statins in the blood could occur as little as 4 hours after drinking a single glass of juice, and last for as long as 72 hours. The strength of this effect can vary from one brand of juice to another, and even between different batches of the same brand. To complicate matters further, the strength of the interaction can vary a great deal from person to person, and there is currently no way to measure this effect. Some studies suggest that small amounts of grapefruit juice, perhaps a few ounces, especially when taken at a different time from the statin, are unlikely to have serious consequences.

The good news is that three other statins—rosuvastatin (Crestor), pravastatin (Pravachol), and fluvastatin (Lescol)— are handled by the body in a different way. There is no interaction between these medications and grapefruit juice, and one of them will almost always be an appropriate substitute. Other ("non-statin") types of cholesterol-lowering medications are also completely unaffected by grapefruit juice.

In summary, while small amounts of grapefruit juice or grapefruit itself are unlikely to cause serious trouble, anyone planning on consuming a significant amount should be using one of the many cholesterol-lowering medications that are not prone to this interaction.

63. Would there be any harm if I decided to stop taking my statin?

You should not stop taking your statin medication unless you are advised to do so by your healthcare provider. However, if you experience muscle pain, tenderness, or weakness that cannot be explained (for example, not due to normal exercise) or any other troublesome side effect and you cannot immediately speak to your healthcare provider or to your pharmacist, you may want to discontinue taking your statin while you try to make contact with your healthcare provider as soon as you can.

64. I have heard that ezetimibe is an alternative to statins that can lower my cholesterol just as well. What is ezetimibe and how does it work?

Statins decrease the amount of cholesterol that the body manufactures. Another source of cholesterol is from certain foods (e.g., eggs). This cholesterol enters the circulation via absorption directly from the food as it passes through the intestine. Blocking intestinal absorption of the cholesterol in food offers another way to prevent cholesterol from accumulating in your body. Ezetimibe (Zetia) is a drug that works in the small intestine to prevent the absorption of cholesterol. Because ezetimibe prevents cholesterol absorption in the gut, its use leads to a reduction in the amount of cholesterol delivered to the liver.

In clinical trials, ezetimibe has been shown to be very effective at lowering LDL cholesterol levels, even when it is prescribed alone. However, it is usually paired with a statin with the aim of lowering LDL cholesterol even further. Your healthcare provider may add ezetimibe to your medication regimen to increase the reduction in your LDL cholesterol without prescribing a higher dose of a statin or prescribing one of the more powerful statins.

65. What are the main side effects of ezetimibe? Is it safe?

Overall, ezetimibe has been found to be a well-tolerated medication. It appears to be a very safe drug. In clinical trials, approximately 4% of patients on ezetimibe complained of diarrhea and 2.5% reported fatigue; this compares with fewer than 4% and 1.5%, respectively, of patients who reported these complaints on placebo (sugar pill). When ezetimibe is given along with a statin, elevations in liver enzymes can occur. Thus you should not be surprised if your healthcare provider tests you for this possibility. Although this side effect occurs more frequently when ezetimibe is added to a statin (in 1.3% of people compared with 0.4% of those on statins alone), it is quite rare.

The other main side effect associated with statins, muscle pain (myopathy), has not been reported with ezetimibe in clinical trials. There have been rare reports of myopathy in the overall population since ezetimibe became available in 2002.

Finally, although interactions between ezetimibe and other drugs you may be taking are rare, patients on cyclosporine (an immunosuppressive medication) should be monitored closely. Taking both cyclosporine and ezetimibe causes the normal blood levels of both drugs to increase.

In 2008, you may have read that the FDA announced that it was reviewing clinical trial data for a possible association between the use of Vytorin—a combination of simvastatin (Zocor) and ezetimibe (Zetia)—and an increased risk of cancer and cancer-related death. After completing its review, however, the FDA announced that it is unlikely that Vytorin or Zetia increase the risk of cancer or cancer-related death.

66. I have heard there is some debate about whether ezetimibe is really beneficial. Is this drug effective?

Ezetimibe is effective in lowering LDL cholesterol levels. This benefit has been shown in many clinical trials and in day-to-day clinical care. Given that more than 20 years of clinical trials and clinical experience have shown that lowering LDL cholesterol has a proven benefit for preventing heart disease events (angina, heart attacks, strokes), simple logic says that ezetimibe should be beneficial for all patients whose LDL cholesterol levels are too high, or who have other risk factors for heart disease.

There is one problem with this logic, however: Most of the statins have been tested by giving some patients a statin and others a placebo. After a few years, more of the patients taking the statin are alive compared to the patients taking the placebo. Thus there can be no question that the statin saved lives. By the time ezetimibe was ready to be tested in patients, however, it was no longer considered ethical to give a patient a placebo that did not contain a cholesterol-lowering drug. Therefore it would be very difficult, and perhaps even unethical, to design a clinical trial to test whether more patients on ezetimibe would be alive compared to patients who were not taking ezetimibe.

What does this mean for you? Strictly speaking, researchers have not proven that ezetimibe will prevent heart attacks, strokes, or death due to cardiovascular disease, although some recent studies suggest it may have a benefit on cardiovascular events. To scientists who take a very strict definition of scientific evidence, this lack of proof means that it is not possible to answer the question whether ezetimibe is beneficial. Additional research to answer the question is in progress.

67. Are there times when I should consider stopping ezetimibe?

Ezetimibe is generally started when a person fails to achieve his or her LDL cholesterol goal even though the individual is following a prescription of diet and statin therapy. By adding ezetimibe to the statin, almost all patients can achieve the LDL cholesterol levels that their healthcare providers tell them they should reach. In addition, for some people, ezetimibe is an appropriate choice because they cannot take a statin (due to statin intolerance). Approximately 25 million people in the United States are taking statins, and as many as 10% experience side effects from these medications (mainly muscle and joint aches). This group of people either cannot tolerate statins at all or can tolerate a statin only at low doses—too low to reach the LDL cholesterol levels they need to reach. For many of these people, ezetimibe will allow them to achieve their LDL cholesterol goal. Given this background, ezetimibe is generally stopped only if a person develops side effects or fails to respond adequately in terms of LDL cholesterol reduction.

68. What is niacin (nicotinic acid) and how does it work?

Niacin, also known as nicotinic acid, is vitamin B3. Your healthcare provider may prescribe niacin as a cholesterol remedy. Niaspan is the only FDA-approved, prescription extended-release niacin formulation for the treatment of lipid disorders. Other formulations of niacin are available as dietary supplements (see Part Nine: Cholesterol-Lowering Dietary Supplements); only prescription niacin is discussed here. When your healthcare provider prescribes a medical dose of niacin to treat your lipids, the dose will usually be 1 g (1000 mg), increasing as soon as you tolerate it to 2 g (2000 mg) daily.

Niacin is a very useful drug. Statins lower your LDL ("bad") cholesterol but have little or no effect on HDL ("good") cholesterol. Niacin, in contrast, has a small-to-medium effect in lowering your LDL cholesterol and a larger effect on increasing your HDL cholesterol. This agent is also beneficial for lowering your triglyceride levels.

It is important to remember that most people with high levels of LDL cholesterol (and/or low levels of HDL cholesterol) do not feel "sick." Therefore, if your healthcare provider has prescribed niacin for you, it is important to continue taking this medication even if you feel well. To get the most benefit from this medicine, you should try to remember to take it at the same time each day, preferably before bedtime, 30 minutes after taking an aspirin or a nonsteroidal anti-inflammatory drug (NSAID), such as ibuprofen (but not acetaminophen). If you forget to take a dose (a "skipped dose"), wait until the next scheduled dosing time and continue with the usual dose; do *not* "double up" the next dose to make up for a missing one.

69. What are the main side effects of niacin?

Niacin is generally a safe and effective drug. In many patients, however, it has a very prominent side effect: facial flushing (a strong sensation of warmth, itching, redness, or tingly feeling under your skin). This effect is especially noticeable when you first begin taking niacin, but will generally disappear over time as you keep taking the medication. In addition, flushing can be made worse if you drink alcohol or hot beverages shortly after you take niacin.

To lessen the chance of side effects such as flushing, avoid consuming alcohol and hot beverages near the time you take niacin. You should consider, and discuss with your healthcare provider, taking a plain (non-enteric-coated) 325 mg aspirin tablet or an NSAID, such as ibuprofen 200 mg, 30 minutes before taking niacin, as this step may help prevent flushing. Taking niacin with foods such as skim milk, low-fat yogurt, or applesauce may also help decrease the risk of flushing.

Niacin can increase blood sugar levels and may cause gout. In addition, a few patients can experience serious allergic reactions to it. If you have any of the following signs of an allergic reaction, you should get emergency medical help immediately: hives, difficulty breathing, or swelling of your face, lips, tongue, or throat. Also call your healthcare provider at once if you have any of these serious side effects:

- Feeling light-headed, fainting
- Fast, pounding, or uneven heartbeats
- Shortness of breath
- Jaundice (yellowing of your skin or eyes)
- Muscle pain, tenderness, or weakness with fever or flu symptoms and dark-colored urine

70. When should I consider stopping taking niacin?

Do not stop taking this medicine unless instructed by your healthcare provider. If niacin is stopped for longer than one missed dose, you may need to return to your original starting dose and gradually increase it again. Consult your healthcare provider or pharmacist for instructions on restarting your niacin if you have not taken your medication for several days.

71. What are fibrates and how do they work?

Because high levels of triglycerides in the circulation are associated with an increased risk of vascular disease, your healthcare provider may want to prescribe a drug treatment if you have high triglyceride levels. Very high triglyceride levels—more than 1000 mg/dL—are also associated with a risk of developing a condition called pancreatitis, in which the pancreas (an organ in the upper abdomen) becomes inflamed due to the high levels of blood fats. Pancreatitis causes severe abdominal pain, nausea, and vomiting and usually requires hospitalization and pain medications. Because it can be very serious, patients require medication to treat the high triglyceride levels.

The drugs most often prescribed for treating high triglycerides, both the moderately high and the very high levels, are known as **fibrates** or fibric acid. Fibrates lower the amount of triglycerides produced by liver cells or increase their removal from the blood. They can also increase HDL cholesterol levels. Three fibrates are available in the United States: fenofibrate (Antara, Lofibra—capsules; Fenoglide, Fibricor, Lipofen, Tricor—tablets),

Fibrates

The oldest class of lipid-lowering drugs, which are useful for treating high triglyceride levels.

fenofibric acid (Trilipix—capsules), and gemfibrozil (Lopid—tablets).

72. What are the main side effects of fibrates?

Fibrate medications are safe and well tolerated. One of the main side effects of fibrates is that they can cause muscle problems similar to the statin medications. When a fibrate (gemfibrozil more than fenofibrate) is used together with a statin, this risk may be further increased; thus this combination should be used with caution. If you are prescribed a fibrate, your healthcare provider will monitor you closely for this side effect, and you should report to your healthcare provider and/or pharmacist if you experience muscle pain, tenderness, or weakness that cannot be explained (for example, not due to normal exercise).

Fibrates have been associated with an increase in gallstones (hard, pebble-sized or larger deposits that form inside the gallbladder). Symptoms of gallstones can include pain in the right upper or middle upper abdomen that occurs within minutes of a meal and may be associated with fever and yellowing of the skin and the whites of the eyes.

73. Are fibrates dangerous? Are they beneficial?

As mentioned in Question 72, fibrate medications are safe and well tolerated, although myopathies and gallstones can occur infrequently. Nevertheless, the evidence supporting the contention that fibrates prevent heart attacks, strokes, and death related to cardiovascular disease is not as clear as for statins. The benefits of fibrates appear to outweigh the risk of side effects, but more research is needed to determine which types of patients are the best candidates for fibrate therapy. Patients who have had pancreatitis due to very high triglyceride levels are almost always treated with fibrates.

74. When should I consider stopping taking my fibrate?

As with most medications, you should not stop taking fibrates unless you have discussed this step with your healthcare practitioner. However, if you experience muscle pain, tenderness, or weakness that cannot be explained (for example, not due to normal exercise) or symptoms associated with gallstones or any other troublesome side effect, and you cannot immediately speak to your healthcare practitioner and or pharmacist, you should discontinue your fibrate medication.

75. What are cholestyramine, colestipol, and colesevelam?

Most of the body's cholesterol, which it needs for healthy cells and metabolism, is produced by the liver. To obtain the building blocks to make this cholesterol, the liver makes compounds called bile acids to break down and digest fats within the gut so that fats and cholesterol can be taken into the body; following this step, the bile acids are normally reabsorbed very efficiently in the small intestine. Bile acids are actually made from cholesterol by the liver. If reabsorption of the bile acids within the gastrointestinal tract is blocked, then the liver is forced to remove more cholesterol, especially LDL ("bad") cholesterol, from the circulation so as to manufacture more bile acid.

Cholestyramine (Prevalite or Questran) is the first FDA-approved member of the class of medications known as "bile acid sequestrants," which act mainly by decreasing the reabsorption of bile acids within the gastrointestinal tract. As a result of this action, cholestyramine and the newer variations of this class of bile acid sequestrants, colestipol (Colestid) and colesevelam (Welchol), can lower LDL cholesterol by approximately 15% to 30% and slightly raise HDL cholesterol by 3% to 5%. These bile acid sequestrants can be prescribed either alone or in combination with a statin to lower LDL cholesterol. Cholestyramine and colestipol are taken orally in powder form added to water two to three times per day with meals. Colestipol is also available in pill form. Colesevelam is prescribed either in pill form taken once or twice per day (maximum of six pills) or in a suspension taken once per day with meals.

The primary benefit of cholestyramine and colestipol use is their safety and effectiveness in lowering LDL cholesterol. These medications have been available for a long time and can be used safely in children and adolescents as well as adults. Because cholestyramine is available in many generic preparations, it is fairly inexpensive. A newly discovered benefit with colesevelam when prescribed for patients with diabetes mellitus is that it lowers glycated hemoglobin (HbA_{1c}), a test of blood sugar control used in patients with diabetes, by 0.5%.

76. What are the major side effects of cholestyramine and the other bile acid sequestrants?

The side-effect profile of these drugs varies according to which drug you are prescribed. The main side effects of cholestyramine and colestipol are gastrointestinal symptoms: development of constipation, abdominal bloating or discomfort, or increased flatulence (gas). Constipation occurs approximately 30% of the time with cholestyramine and colestipol, but only rarely becomes severe enough to cause fecal (stool) impaction in the large intestine (bowel obstruction). Constipation can be prevented or treated with increased intake of fluids and dietary fiber, use of fiber supplements (such as Metamucil, Citracel, or Benefiber), or use of stool softeners (such as Colace).

Cholestyramine, colestipol, and colesevelam can raise your triglyceride levels significantly if you have preexisting elevated triglycerides. In addition, when cholestyramine is prescribed in combination with a statin, in rare cases liver enzyme levels can become elevated. In addition, cholestyramine and colestipol can reduce the absorption of other medications and fat-soluble vitamins such as vitamins A, D, E, or K, thereby decreasing their effectiveness. This problem can potentially be avoided by taking the other medications or vitamins either 1 hour before or 4 hours after you take cholestyramine. The newest member of the bile acid sequestrant class, colesevelam, is less likely to cause these side effects and, therefore, is better tolerated. Unlike cholestyramine and colestipol, colesevelam also seems less likely to interfere with absorption of other medications.

77. When should I consider stopping taking a bile acid sequestrant?

Reasons for the immediate discontinuation of cholestyramine and other bile acid sequestrants include development of an allergic reaction; intolerable abdominal bloating, gas, or pain; severe or persistent constipation that is not improved with the use of stool softeners or fiber supplements; fecal impaction; or bowel obstruction. Considerations for probable discontinuation of these medications might be raised with the occurrence of worsening liver function tests, a significant increase in serum triglyceride levels, or concerns about reduced effectiveness of other medications due to the interference of drug absorption as a result of cholestyramine or colestipol use.

78. How do you decide when to combine cholesterol medicines?

In calculating the risk for developing cardiovascular disease, higher levels of LDL cholesterol and triglycerides result in higher risk, whereas higher levels of HDL cholesterol are generally protective. In patients at high cardiovascular risk, it may be appropriate to continue treatment until all three factors have reached their ideal levels. A statin is usually the first choice for medical therapy because of the statins' long safety record and great effectiveness in reducing LDL cholesterol, though they have only a modest impact on triglycerides and HDL cholesterol. When the highest appropriate dose of a statin fails to lower the LDL cholesterol and triglycerides to normal, or if a patient needs something to increase his or her HDL cholesterol, combination therapy may be necessary.

Any combination of two or more cholesterol-lowering medications is permitted, although gemfibrozil should not generally be combined with a statin. As always, when multiple medications of any kind are used, additional monitoring may be required. Physicians have been using various combinations of blood pressure-lowering medications for many years; it should not be surprising that the same approach may often be necessary for cholesterol-lowering medications.

Your healthcare provider may prescribe a "fixed-dose" drug combination, which means that you have to take only one pill that contains two drugs. Fixed-dose combination lipid-lowering drugs available in the United States include these products:

- Vytorin (simvastatin + ezetimibe)
- Advicor (extended-release niacin + lovastatin)
- Simcor (extended-release niacin + simvastatin)

Another combination therapy that you may come across is a brand called Caduet, which combines a statin cholesterol-lowering drug (atorvastatin) with a blood-pressure-lowering drug (amlodipine).

Paul's comment:

I had been taking rosuvastatin for a while and my LDL (bad cholesterol) was nice and low. My doctor was not satisfied because my triglycerides were a little high and my HDL (good cholesterol) was still very low. He added niacin and after a number of months, my triglycerides were low and my HDL began to increase. Now he says that my overall "profile" is ideal, and we are both happy.

79. Will cholesterol medications damage my liver?

With more than 20 years of experience and more than 25 million Americans taking statins, it is clear that the likelihood of serious liver problems (liver failure or death) with use of cholesterol medications is very low. Most authorities estimate that the rate of liver problems in persons taking statins is 1 to 2 per 1 million patients—a rate that is similar to that for other commonly used medications, including various antibiotics. Mild abnormalities of liver blood tests can occur with any of the statins (less than 1% of the time and more frequently at higher doses). These issues are not considered to indicate liver damage or abnormal function. According to studies, approximately 70% of the abnormalities return to the normal range even when treatment is continued. For this reason, according to the National Lipid Association's Statin Safety Task Force, routine monitoring of liver blood tests is not really necessary. That said, most physicians continue to check liver function tests periodically (about every 6 to 12 months) in patients taking statins.

Among the other cholesterol-lowering medications, ezetimibe, fibrates, and omega-3 fish oils (see Part Nine: Cholesterol-Lowering Dietary Supplements) are not believed to have significant effects on the liver. Niacin infrequently causes liver problems, which can be reversed by stopping niacin or using lower doses. Severe liver damage has been reported rarely with niacin, mostly related to the use of nonprescription slow-release preparations available as over-the-counter supplements.

As with everything in medicine, it is always necessary to weigh the benefits associated with a medication against the possible risks. The benefits of cholesterol-altering medications, particularly statins, which can dramatically reduce heart attacks and strokes, greatly outweigh the rare possibility of a serious liver problem.

Stephanie's comment:

You always hear "people" talk about cholesterol medication being bad for your liver, but it's true that I have never heard of anyone having a problem. My doctor assured me of the medication's safety, and said that even though it was not necessary, he would be happy to check my liver blood tests periodically if I would prefer.

80. How long do I have to take my cholesterol-lowering medications?

Humans begin to develop atherosclerosis of their blood vessels at a very young age. If they are overweight as teenagers, then they are already beginning to develop fatty deposits in their arteries. As a result, dyslipidemia (abnormal amounts of LDL cholesterol, HDL cholesterol, or triglycerides in your blood) is a lifelong disease. This means that once you have been diagnosed with dyslipidemia, you will need to pay attention to changing your "lipid metabolism" for the rest of your life. Of course, the best way to ensure that you have healthy blood vessels is to make sure that you do not smoke, overeat, or consume a diet too high in fatty calories, and that you maintain adequate levels of activity. For more on these issues, see the parts of this book on managing your cholesterol by diet (Part Six) and physical exercise (Part Seven).

For many people, diet and exercise are not enough to correct for disorders of their lipid metabolism, and they need to take lipid-modifying medications. Some of the effects of these medications may occur rather quickly, whereas other benefits become more pronounced over time. At first, a statin (or other medication) may actually improve the healthy functioning of your arteries. Over a longer period of time, cholesterol-altering medications will prevent further build-up of cholesterol deposits within the artery, and in some cases they may even reduce the degree of a cholesterol deposition. This effect accumulates over years, so it makes sense that the longer you take the medication, the better.

81. Can I stop my medications when my lipid "numbers" improve?

This question is closely related to Question 80. Generally, if your cholesterol levels improve on the medication but nothing else (for example, diet, exercise habits, smoking) has changed, your numbers would be expected to return to their pre-medication levels soon after you discontinue the medication. In such a case, the medication simply controls the problem; it does not cure it.

There is no question that lifestyle changes can have dramatic effects on all lipid parameters, lowering the LDL ("bad") cholesterol and triglycerides, as well as raising the HDL ("good") cholesterol. If your numbers eventually reach levels that your healthcare provider believes are healthy, considering your overall health, age, and other risk factors—and especially your general lifestyle and diet—it may be possible to cut back or taper down your lipid medications.

Lifestyle changes may even allow some people to stop their medications. This possibility should be a strong incentive to augment your medications with a real dedication to modifying your diet and increasing your overall activity levels so as to achieve the healthy lipid numbers that your medications are trying to achieve. Until then, you should remember that statins, and most other lipid-modifying medications, have a record for being among the safest medications available. As long as your lipid levels are unhealthy, you should be taking your medications. If you have familial hypercholesterolemia, you will need medication even if you have a healthy lifestyle.

David's comment:

I asked my doctor if I would be able to stop the medication if I adopted a healthy diet and began to exercise. He said that it might be possible—it was worth a try. Of course, I didn't, but after 2 years, my friend Rich had a small heart attack, and we both decided to get healthy. After 6 months I lost 25 pounds and my cholesterol was so low that my doctor and I agreed to discontinue the medication, with close follow-up.

82. Are there any medicines that will make my cholesterol worse?

Any medicine that raises LDL cholesterol would be considered to be making your cholesterol worse. Likewise, because the ratio of HDL to LDL ("good to bad") cholesterol is also a predictor of risk for cardiovascular disease, any medicine that lowers HDL would be considered to be making things worse.

There are a few medicines that raise LDL cholesterol:

- The class known as anabolic steroids (androgens), including testosterone, can raise LDL. These agents are used for several disorders, most commonly low testosterone levels in men. They also include the steroids that are frequently abused by professional and amateur athletes.

- Retinoids, which are used in skin conditions such as psoriasis and severe acne, can raise LDL cholesterol.

- Progestins, especially those used in birth control pills, can increase LDL cholesterol. Because they are often used in combination with estrogen, however, the net effect on the overall "good to bad ratio" may be negligible.

- Cyclosporine and other immunosuppressants used in organ transplant recipients require that cholesterol levels be monitored carefully. This is also true for the protease inhibitors used to treat HIV infection.

- Corticosteroids, such as those used in asthma and certain rheumatologic conditions, generally cause a mild rise in LDL cholesterol.

- The diabetes drugs known as thiazolidinediones (TZDs) such as pioglitazone (Actos), the only TZD generally available in the United States at present, and rosiglitazone (Avandia; use restricted) can increase LDL cholesterol.

- The diuretic (water pill) known as hydrochlorothiazide, which is used as a blood pressure medication, can increase LDL cholesterol levels mildly (by approximately 15%) in some patients.

Many of the same medications mentioned as increasing LDL cholesterol (androgens most notably, as well as progestins and retinoids) can also reduce HDL cholesterol.

Some of the older beta blockers used in heart disease, such as propranolol, and the phenothiazines, which are used in various psychiatric conditions, can also reduce levels of HDL cholesterol to a significant degree. However, both corticosteroids and pioglitazone also tend to raise HDL cholesterol, so this effect may cancel out the negative impact on LDL cholesterol.

83. Are there medications that can make my triglyceride levels worse?

Many drugs may have a negative effect on your triglyceride levels, including these:

- Oral forms of estrogen, including birth control pills.
- Retinoids.
- Corticosteroids.
- Medications used for HIV infection, especially protease inhibitors.
- Phenothiazines and other antipsychotic drugs.
- Older beta blockers such as propranolol (Inderal), atenolol (Tenormin), and metoprolol (Lopressor). Be sure to mention to your healthcare provider if you are taking a beta blocker.
- Hydrochlorothiazide.

Other agents that can increase triglycerides include tamoxifen, which is used in the treatment of breast cancer. Cyclophosphamide, which is used in the treatment of many types of cancer, has the same effect. The bile acid sequestrants—cholestyramine, colestipol, and colesevelam—are an interesting case. While they are helpful in lowering LDL cholesterol, they are also known to increase triglycerides, which limits their usefulness in many patients.

84. What is prescription fish oil and what are its uses?

High doses of the long-chain fatty acids, EPA and DHA, can lower triglyceride levels. One prescription form of fish oil in a fixed-dose capsule, Lovaza, has been approved to lower triglycerides. The dose consists of four capsules per day, which can lower triglyceride levels by approximately 30%. This medication does not have any effect on cholesterol levels. The main side effects are forms of stomach upset such as diarrhea and burping. The prescription fish oil capsules are more purified than most over-the-counter fish oil/omega-3 supplements and, therefore, contain a higher amount of EPA and DHA.

PART NINE

Cholesterol– Lowering Dietary Supplements

Should I consider taking dietary supplements?

What are stanols and sterols?

Does garlic lower cholesterol?

More . . .

85. Should I consider taking dietary supplements?

You may have been exercising and eating a healthier diet, and you might wonder whether adding a cholesterol-lowering dietary supplement to your diet could help reduce your cholesterol further. Only a few supplements have been proven to reduce cholesterol, but you and your healthcare provider might consider that these cholesterol-lowering supplements could help you. You should start taking them only after discussion with your healthcare provider, especially because dietary supplements may interfere with the effects of prescription medications you are taking.

86. Are dietary supplements safe?

In the United States, manufacturers and distributors of dietary supplements do not need approval from the Food and Drug Administration to sell them, provided the ingredients were approved for use before 1994. The Current Good Manufacturing Practices (CGMPs) are rules established by the FDA to ensure the purity, quality, and strength of a supplement. The newest regulations are intended to ensure that dietary supplements do not have wrong ingredients, too much or too little of the dietary ingredient, improper labeling and packaging, and contamination problems such as bacteria, natural toxins, pesticides, lead, glass, or other substances.

The FDA requires all ingredients in the capsules to be listed on a product label, including capsule additives such as gelatins and starch, as well as preservatives and dyes. These rules give the dietary supplement industry clear expectations, but it is the responsibility of the FDA to audit and enforce these new regulations. However, supplements are not subject to the same scrutiny and high standards that apply to prescription medications. Notably, contamination and false labeling have been found with some supplements.

Because manufacturers and distributors do not need FDA approval to sell their dietary supplements, there is no government-developed list of manufacturers, distributors, or the dietary supplement products they sell. Some supplements have been tested and compared by ConsumerLab.com, which issues its reports online (see the Appendix for more on this organization). The information on this site can help guide you if you decide you want to take supplements.

The supplements discussed in Part Nine are just a few of the wide variety on sale that claim to be beneficial for your cholesterol and triglycerides. They are sold under many different names.

87. Should I take fish oil?

Fish oil has been found to protect the arteries by decreasing inflammation. It reduces the tendency for blood clots to form, and it also lowers triglyceride levels when given at adequate doses. Your diet should provide most of your fish oil intake, but for patients with coronary artery disease, the AHA advises a 1 g daily supplement of omega-3 fatty acids, which should contain both EPA (eicosapentaenoic acid) and DHA (docosahexaenoic acid), as an alternative. This supplement may be taken after consultation with your healthcare provider.

One prescription form of fish oil in a fixed-dose capsule has been approved to lower triglycerides. Your healthcare provider will prescribe fish oil at the appropriate dose if you have high triglycerides. This issue is dealt with in Question 84 (in Part Eight: Managing Your Cholesterol with Medications). Over-the-counter fish oil varies widely in the amount of EPA and DHA in each capsule from each supplier. It is also sold as a liquid. You may experience a fishy aftertaste in your mouth after taking any fish oil supplement, and all of these supplements can cause bad breath, gas, nausea, vomiting, or diarrhea.

88. Isn't there a risk of poisoning by mercury and other contaminants in fish oil?

This is a valid concern, as independent studies performed by organizations such as ConsumerLab.com have found that some brands of fish oil contain rancid fatty acids that can harm your health. Fish from all parts of the world may be contaminated to some degree by mercury and other industrial pollutants, so you should be very careful that the fish oil you buy is a validated brand.

89. Should I take vitamin E?

Vitamin E is a fat-soluble vitamin that is found naturally in some foods, but can also be taken as a dietary supplement. Vitamin E has not been shown to alter cholesterol or triglyceride levels and should not be used for this purpose. It has antioxidant properties and in animal experiments has been shown to reduce oxidation of lipoproteins, which is important in reducing the development of coronary heart disease. However, human studies have not shown that vitamin E reduces the risk of coronary heart disease when compared with placebo (sugar pills).

90. Should I take vitamin B supplements?

Vitamin B consists of eight water-soluble vitamins that play important roles in the maintenance of normal cellular functions that support body metabolism, the immune and nervous systems, and red blood cell growth. A properly balanced diet of whole foods is a good source of B vitamins. With the exception of vitamin B3 (niacin), as discussed in Part Eight: Managing Your Cholesterol with Medications, B vitamins have not been shown to alter cholesterol or triglyceride levels and should not be used for this purpose.

Elevations in blood levels of homocysteine (an amino acid that acts as a building block for making proteins) have been identified as a risk factor for coronary heart disease. Supplementation with folic acid (vitamin B_9), pyridoxine (vitamin B_6), or cyanocobalamin (vitamin B_{12}) does lower blood levels of homocysteine, but has not been shown to reduce the risk for coronary heart disease.

91. Will taking over-the-counter niacin (nicotinic acid) improve my cholesterol?

A number of niacin supplements are available as over-the-counter products. One is Slo-Niacin, a tablet that you take twice a day in the morning or evening. It releases the niacin into your body slowly throughout the day, thereby reducing—although not completely eliminating—the flushing effect associated with niacin. However, the dosages sold are lower than those recommended for the form of niacin available by prescription, which is the dose shown to be beneficial for cholesterol (see Part Eight:

Managing Your Cholesterol with Medications). You should use high dosages of over-the-counter niacin supplements only with the supervision of your healthcare provider. The niacin that your healthcare provider prescribes is also a controlled-release product that reduces flushing.

92. Will taking over-the-counter "no flush" or "flush free" niacin improve my cholesterol safely?

The niacin (nicotinic acid) that you get by prescription from your healthcare provider reduces LDL ("bad") cholesterol and triglycerides and raises HDL ("good") cholesterol, but it may cause flushing (see Part Eight: Managing Your Cholesterol with Medications). Some over-the-counter dietary supplements claim to improve your cholesterol in the same way as niacin without the flushing side effect, but there is little scientific evidence to support that claim.

Niacinamide or **nicotinamide** is part of the vitamin B group, like niacin. However, niacinamide has very little or no effect on cholesterol. It is often mistaken for a good alternative to niacin because it does not cause flushing. Niacinamide and niacin can be considered to be equivalent only for the purposes of nutritional supplementation (at low doses, not intended to treat cholesterol).

Inositol hexaniacinate, also known as inositol nicotinate, consists of six niacin molecules cross-linked to an inositol molecule. There is little scientific evidence that inositol hexaniacinate improves cholesterol at lower doses and the safety profile of inositol hexaniacinate has not been studied.

Niacinamide (nicotinamide)

A member of the vitamin B group that has very little or no effect on cholesterol.

93. *What is red yeast rice?*

Red yeast rice is a traditional Chinese cuisine and medicinal agent made by fermenting rice with the yeast *Monascus purpureus*. Scientific studies in China and the United States have reported that red yeast rice can significantly reduce LDL ("bad") cholesterol and total cholesterol in humans. Red yeast rice contains naturally occurring statin-like substances called monacolins. The main one, monacolin K, is the same compound as lovastatin, the first statin ever approved in the United States (see Part Eight: Managing Your Cholesterol with Medications). Products containing lovastatin are considered to be "new drugs" and may not be legally marketed without approval by the FDA. In 2007, the FDA discovered that a number of red yeast rice supplements contained monacolin K/lovastatin. However, recent analyses of a number of red yeast rice formulations currently available showed that they contained varying amounts of monacolin K/lovastatin, so there is no way to know what level or quality of lovastatin might be present in each red yeast rice supplement. More information about red yeast rice supplements and what they contain is available from ConsumerLabs.com (see the Appendix at the end of the book).

94. *What are stanols and sterols?*

Stanols and **sterols**, also called phytostanols and phytosterols, are very similar to cholesterol but occur in plants rather than in animals. Their cholesterol-lowering effects were first reported in the 1950s. Research has shown that plant stanols (which are usually modified into stanol esters) can help to lower cholesterol in people with

Stanols
Phytostanols; compounds that are very similar to cholesterol but occur in plants rather than in animals. Their cholesterol-lowering effects were first reported in the 1950s.

Sterols
Phytosterols; compounds that are very similar to cholesterol but occur in plants rather than in animals. Their cholesterol-lowering effects were first reported in the 1950s.

normal or mildly to moderately raised levels. Stanols and sterols have been incorporated into various food products and herbal supplements. Margarines that contain stanols or sterols will indicate that fact on the product label.

Both sterols and stanols compete with cholesterol for absorption from the gastrointestinal tract and lower blood levels of cholesterol from 10% to 15% when taken in large amounts (1 to 2 g) on a daily basis. Current research suggests that the use of these products is safe, but there is still some debate about whether they interfere with the absorption of nutrients in the intestine. The most tested sterol and stanol are beta-sitosterol and sitostanol, respectively.

95. What is flaxseed oil?

Flaxseed oil

An oil obtained from the seed of the flax plant (*Linum usitatissimum*), an edible seed/grain. It contains omega-3 fatty acids, but does not appear to lower blood triglyceride levels very much.

Flaxseed oil is obtained from the seed of the flax plant (*Linum usitatissimum*), an edible seed/grain. Flaxseed oil contains omega-3 acids, which are considered essential fatty acids (humans must get them from food for good health). The fatty acids that can lower blood triglyceride levels are eicosapentaenoic acid (EPA) and docosahexaenoic acid (DHA), which are present in fish oil. However, a large percentage of the essential fatty acid content of flaxseed oil (approximately 60%) is in the form of alpha-linolenic acid (ALA). The human body can convert this fatty acid to EPA and DHA, but only in very small amounts. In several well-designed human studies, flaxseed oil did not lower blood triglyceride levels very much, so it should not be used for this purpose. However, ALA may have other beneficial effects on the heart, such as a reduction in inflammation.

96. What is policosanol?

Policosanol is a mixture of waxy substances usually manufactured from sugarcane. It contains approximately 60% octacosanol, along with many related chemicals. In some cases, the terms "octacosanol" and "policosanol" are used interchangeably. Octacosanol is also found in wheat germ oil, rice bran, vegetable oils, alfalfa, and various animal products.

Policosanol was originally developed in Cuba and results from the early studies conducted by investigators in Cuba were very promising. Policosanol was reported to reduce LDL cholesterol by approximately 24%. On this basis, policosanol has been approved as a treatment for high cholesterol in approximately two dozen countries, most of them in Latin America. Independent human studies conducted in the United States and Europe did not find policosanol to lower LDL cholesterol more than placebo (sugar pill). Thus this supplement should not be used for the purpose of lowering blood cholesterol levels.

Due to political and patent issues, the Cuban sugarcane policosanol has not been widely available in the United States. Products sold in the U.S. market as "policosanol" are generally derived from beeswax or wheat germ. Studies of these products have also shown no beneficial effect on cholesterol.

97. Does garlic lower cholesterol?

Some studies have shown that garlic produces a moderate, short-term reduction in total cholesterol in the range of 4% to 12%, including decreases in triglycerides and LDL ("bad") cholesterol. Garlic may also slow the development of atherosclerosis. However, most studies have shown no benefit of garlic on cholesterol. Because of the varying results, it is not recommended as a cholesterol-lowering agent in guidelines.

Garlic is sold as pills that contain garlic powder. For those interested in using garlic in their diet, raw garlic that is crushed, chopped, or chewed is most effective. Cooked garlic is less powerful, and stomach acid blocks the benefit of powdered garlic unless it is in an enteric-coated pill. A well-known side effect of garlic is unpleasant breath odor. Even "odorless" garlic tablets produce an offensive smell in as many as 50% of people who use it.

98. I drink green tea because I believe it's really good for me. I've heard that it can lower high cholesterol—is this true?

The health benefits reported with green tea are usually attributed to the high concentration of powerful antioxidants called polyphenols in the tea. These antioxidants are believed to be capable of removing free radicals—damaging compounds in the body that change cells, alter DNA, and cause cell death. Antioxidants can neutralize free radicals and may reduce or prevent some of the damage they cause.

Several studies have shown that people who drank green tea had lower total cholesterol levels than people who did not drink the same tea. In another study, green tea appeared to lower LDL cholesterol. Studies in animals suggested that the polyphenols in green tea might block the intestinal absorption of cholesterol and promote its excretion from the body. Studies in overseas populations have concluded that green tea might prevent atherosclerosis. However, after reviewing the evidence, the FDA concluded that there was no credible evidence that green tea or green tea extract could reduce the risk of heart disease.

99. Can chelation therapy improve my cholesterol numbers?

Chelation therapy has been used to treat poisoning from heavy metals such as lead or mercury. An amino acid called EDTA (ethylenediamine tetraacetic acid), when given intravenously, will bind with these toxins and reduce their levels in the body by elimination through the urine. EDTA also binds or connects with calcium in the body—and calcium is one component found in coronary artery plaques. For more than 30 years, some people have sought an alternative treatment to traditional medical therapy for the plaque build-up in the coronary arteries. Although chelation therapy has been effective in removing heavy metals from the body, it has not been proven to remove the fatty calcified plaques in the coronary arteries.

A review of the scientific literature on chelation therapy revealed that the following organizations do **not** support treatment with chelation therapy for coronary artery disease: the American Heart Association; the Food and Drug Administration; the American College of Physicians; the National Heart, Lung, and Blood Institute; the American Medical Association; and the American College of Cardiology.

100. Where can I find more information about managing my cholesterol?

The Appendix that follows lists a selection of online resources for more information about managing your cholesterol.

CHOLESTEROL-LOWERING DIETARY SUPPLEMENTS

Cholesterol and Cardiovascular Disease Risk

Government Agencies

Centers for Disease Control and Prevention (CDC)

http://www.cdc.gov/cholesterol/index.htm
High Cholesterol: Understanding Your Risks
Cholesterol home page of the CDC. Links to learning about
cholesterol and facts and statistics about cholesterol.

Food and Drug Administration (FDA)

http://www.fda.gov/forconsumers/byaudience/forwomen/
ucm118595.htm
High Cholesterol—Medicines To Help You

National Heart, Lung, and Blood Institute (NHLBI)

http://www.nhlbi.nih.gov/health/index.htm
Home page of the public web site of the National Heart, Lung,
and Blood Institute (NHLBI), linking to health information,
publications, web sites, and web applications.

http://www.nhlbi.nih.gov/health/public/heart/index.htm#chol
Page of the NHLBI's web site dedicated to heart and vascular
disease. It contains a list of downloadable guides and fact sheets
about cholesterol.

http://www.nhlbi.nih.gov/health/public/heart/chol/wyntk.htm
Blood Cholesterol: What You Need to Know
Home page for public information about the National Cholesterol
Education Program (NCEP) Third Report on the Detection,
Evaluation, and Treatment of High Blood Cholesterol in Adults
(Adult Treatment Panel III [ATP III]).

http://www.nhlbi.nih.gov/about/ncep/index.htm
National Cholesterol Education Program
Raising awareness and understanding about high blood cholesterol
as a risk factor for CHD and the benefits of lowering cholesterol
levels as a means of preventing CHD.

Medical and Health Associations

American College of Cardiology Foundation (ACCF)
http://www.cardiosmart.org/
Cardiosmart
Home page of the consumer information service of the ACCF.

http://www.cardiosmart.org/conditioncenters/ctt.aspx?id=3136
Cholesterol Condition Center
ACCF's home page links to information about cholesterol, questions to ask your cardiologist, what your doctor is reading, news, and videos.

American Heart Association (AHA)
http://www.heart.org/
Home page of the American Heart Association's web site for patients.

http://www.heart.org/HEARTORG/Conditions/Cholesterol/
CholestrolATH_UCM_001089_SubHomePage.jsp
Cholesterol Tools and Resources
Home page of the AHA's patient site with links to pages on understanding cholesterol and the risks associated with it, monitoring cholesterol, prevention and treatment, and tools and resources on heart, vascular, and blood diseases.

For Women
http://www.goredforwomen.org/index.aspx
Go Red for Women
Home page of the AHA's health information site specifically for women. Includes information and advice on managing cholesterol and other cardiovascular disease risk factors.

National Lipid Association (NLA)
http://www.learnyourlipids.com/
Learn Your Lipids
An overview of the different types of lipids and information about why it is important to have lipid levels in a healthy range and how to achieve those levels. Also a link to "Find a Lipidologist."

Hospitals

Mayo Clinic
http://www.mayoclinic.com/health/high-blood-cholesterol/DS00178
MayoClinic.com
'High cholesterol' with links to other parts of the health information site, questions and answers, and multimedia.

Specialist Groups

Children
American Academy of Pediatrics
http://www.healthychildren.org/
HealthyChildren
Web site of the American Academy of Pediatrics. The site includes information on cholesterol in children and adolescents and advice on how to reduce fat and cholesterol in children's diet.

Familial Hypercholesterolemia
National Human Genome Research Institute
http://www.genome.gov/25520184
Learning about Familial Hypercholesterolemia
Home page with links to other resources.

Commercial Consumer Health Information Providers

About.com.Cholesterol

http://cholesterol.about.com/

Advice on cholesterol management, testing, treatment, and diet plans. Features blogs and discussion groups.

WebMD

http://www.webmd.com/cholesterol-management/default.htm

Cholesterol Management Health Center

How to manage your cholesterol. Comprehensive site from the U.S. provider of health information services.

Diet

American Dietetic Association

http://www.eatright.org/Public/

Watch and Learn Video Library

In addition, click on the For the Public tab to navigate a wealth of nutrition information. For personalized nutrition information, please click on the tab "Find a Registered Dietitian."

American Heart Association

http://www.heart.org/HEARTORG/GettingHealthy/
NutritionCenter/Nutrition-Center_UCM_001188_SubHomePage.js

Nutrition Center

Advice on diet. For example, how many calories you need to consume each day and how much sugar, fat, and protein to consume. It also defines the difference between good fats and bad fats.

United States Department of Agriculture (USDA) Center for Nutrition Policy and Promotion
http://www.cnpp.usda.gov/dietaryguidelines.htm
Dietary Guidelines for Americans

http://www.cnpp.usda.gov/DGAs2010-DGACReport.htm
Report of the Dietary Guidelines Advisory Committee on the Dietary Guidelines for Americans, 2010
Download the latest, science-based nutritional and dietary guidance for the general public aimed at promoting "health and to reduce the risk for major chronic diseases through diet and physical activity."

http://www.choosemyplate.gov
The food guidance system that translates nutritional recommendations into the kinds and amounts of food to eat each day.

Dietary Supplements

ConsumerLab.com
http://www.consumerlab.com/
ConsumerLab.com provides independent test results and information about health and nutrition products. CL also conducts an annual Survey of Vitamin and Supplement Users. Recent reports include including red yeast rice and omega-3 fish oil supplements.

Slow-Niacin Dietary Supplement
http://www.slo-niacin.com/about-slo-niacin
Upsher-Smith web site about *Slo-Niacin*.

Physical Activity

American Heart Association
http://www.heart.org/HEARTORG/GettingHealthy/PhysicalActivity/Physical-Activity_UCM_001080_SubHomePage.jsp
Get Started
How to get started on a physical exercise program.

American College of Sports Medicine
http://www.acsm.org/AM/Template.cfm?Section=Home_Page&
TEMPLATE=CM/HTMLDisplay.cfm&CONTENTID=7764
Home page. Download the *Physical Activity and Public Health Guidelines*. Links to information about starting an exercise program.

Drugs

WebMD
Drugs and Medications Information Center
http://www.webmd.com/drugs/index-drugs.aspx

A

Angina: Deep or poorly localized chest or arm pain that occurs when the heart is not receiving enough oxygen. Severe angina, or angina with little stress or exertion, is referred to as "unstable" and may signify an impending heart attack.

Apolipoprotein (apoprotein): A protein found on the surface of a lipoprotein.

Apolipoprotein B (apoB): The apolipoprotein associated with LDL cholesterol and other lipoproteins that are involved with atherosclerosis.

Apolipoprotein A-I (apoA-I): A protein found on HDL particles.

Atherosclerosis: The process in which excess cholesterol in the body's circulation is deposited into cells in the artery walls, where it gradually forms a fatty deposit called a plaque.

B

Blood clot (thrombus): Accumulation of material in a blood vessel that either stops bleeding or stops blood flow through the artery or vein.

Body mass index (BMI): A frequently employed index of obesity, expressed as weight in kilograms (kg) divided by the square of height in meters (m^2); BMI = kg/m^2.

C

Cardiovascular risk factor: Anything that increases the chance of an individual developing cardiovascular disease. It may be either modifiable—that is, things or behaviors that a person can change (e.g., smoking)—or nonmodifiable—that is, things that a person cannot change (e.g., age, family history).

Cholesterol: A wax-like, fatty substance that forms part of cell membranes and used in the production of certain vitamins and hormones, such as vitamin D, cortisol, estrogen, and testosterone. Cholesterol is produced in the liver, which can make all the cholesterol that the body needs. It also enters the body from foods of animal origin, as well as foods that come from animals and products made with these ingredients.

Claudication: Leg pain caused by peripheral artery disease, in which there is not enough blood flow to an area such as the lower legs. Pain often occurs with exertion such as walking or climbing stairs and is relieved by resting.

D

Diabetes mellitus: A disorder caused by disturbance of the normal action of insulin (a hormone responsible for lowering blood sugar) and characterized by high blood sugar levels. This condition is associated with high blood sugar levels resulting from the body's inability to use blood glucose for energy.

Dyslipidemia: Any disorder of levels of cholesterol and triglycerides including high levels of LDL ("bad" cholesterol), high levels of triglycerides, and low levels of HDL ("good" cholesterol).

F

Familial hypercholesterolemia: An inherited condition characterized by abnormally high cholesterol levels in the blood. Affected individuals are unable to process LDL cholesterol properly, and they are at increased risk for coronary heart disease.

Fibrates: The oldest class of lipid-lowering drugs, which are useful for treating high triglyceride levels.

Flaxseed oil: An oil obtained from the seed of the flax plant (*Linum usitatissimum*), an edible seed/grain. It contains omega-3 fatty acids, but does not appear to lower blood triglyceride levels very much.

H

High-density lipoprotein (HDL) cholesterol: HDL cholesterol is called the "good" cholesterol because high levels are often associated with a decreased risk of CHD.

HMG-CoA reductase inhibitors: Medications that lower the level of LDL cholesterol and are the most commonly used medications to treat high cholesterol levels.

Hydroxymethylglutaryl coenzyme-A reductase (HMG-CoA reductase): One of the body's key enzymes, which works in the liver to produce cholesterol.

Hypercholesterolemia (hyperlipidemia): High cholesterol; also known as hyperlipemia or hyperlipoproteinemia.

Hypertension: High blood pressure. The force of blood through and against the walls of arteries causes blood pressure to rise and fall during the day. If blood pressure remains elevated, it is diagnosed as high blood pressure or hypertension.

Hypertriglyceridemia: High triglyceride levels in the blood.

I

Insulin: A hormone responsible for lowering blood sugar.

Ischemia: A decrease of blood flow to a part of the body due to narrowing or blockage of a blood vessel. This can affect the heart muscle causing angina or a heart attack; the legs, causing claudication; or the brain causing a TIA or stroke.

Isolated low HDL cholesterol: The situation in which HDL cholesterol is low, but other lipoproteins are at normal levels.

L

Lipid: Any of a group of fats, or fat-like substances, oils, and waxes, that are insoluble in water, and that serve as building blocks and energy sources for the body.

Lipid profile: A series of tests measuring total cholesterol, LDL cholesterol, HDL cholesterol, and triglycerides.

Lipidologist: Someone who specializes in the treatment of cholesterol problems.

Lipoprotein: Any of a group of protein-covered fat particles that help to transport cholesterol and triglycerides around the body. The four basic classes are high-density, low-density, and very-low-density lipoproteins, and chylomicrons.

Lipoprotein(a): Lp(a); a lipoprotein particle similar to LDL with an attached protein. Elevated blood plasma levels are positively correlated with coronary heart disease.

Low-density lipoprotein (LDL) cholesterol: "Bad" cholesterol. A lipoprotein that carries cholesterol to the blood vessels supplying the tissues where it can build up in the artery walls and cause atherosclerosis.

M

The metabolic syndrome: A syndrome consisting of three or more risk factors that increase the likelihood of developing heart disease: abdominal obesity (waist circumference) greater than 40 inches for men or greater than 35 inches for women; triglycerides greater than 150 mg/dL; HDL cholesterol less than 40 mg/dL in men and less than 50 mg/dL in women; blood pressure greater than 130/85 mm Hg; fasting glucose greater than 110 mg/dL; or taking medications for any of these conditions. Weight loss can improve all of these risk factors.

Myalgia: Muscle aches or weakness that occurs without changes in muscle cells.

Myocardial infarction: Heart attack or death of heart muscle. In severe cases, myocardial infarction can lead to sudden death.

Myopathy: Any disease of muscles. Symptoms include limb and respiratory weakness. Myopathy can result from endocrine disorders, metabolic disorders, infection, or inflammation of the muscle.

Myositis: Muscle symptoms with an increase in blood tests of muscle enzymes indicating inflammation.

N

Niacin: A B vitamin (B3) that is very effective at lowering triglycerides and raising HDL cholesterol.

Niacinamide (nicotinamide): A member of the vitamin B group that has very little or no effect on cholesterol.

Non-HDL cholesterol: A measurement calculated by subtracting HDL cholesterol from total cholesterol; it includes all forms of cholesterol known to form plaque in the arteries.

O

Omega-3 fatty acids: Unsaturated fatty acids that are present in marine animal fats and some vegetable oils.

P

Plaque: Buildup of cholesterol and fatty deposits in the arteries that may gradually narrow the space in the arteries available for the blood to flow to the affected organ.

Plaque rupture: A situation in which a plaque has part of its covering come off exposing the fatty material underneath. This can lead to a blood clot and blockage of the artery containing the plaque.

R

Red yeast rice: A supplement that can lower total cholesterol and LDL cholesterol.

Reverse cholesterol transport: An action of HDL involving transfer of cholesterol from cells back to the liver for removal.

Rhabdomyolysis: A creatine kinase (CK) level greater than 10,000 IU/L, or myopathy plus end organ damage indicated by a significant elevation of serum creatinine.

S

Stanols: Phytostanols; compounds that are very similar to cholesterol but occur in plants rather than in animals. Their cholesterol-lowering effects were first reported in the 1950s.

Statin: A general term for an HMG-CoA reductase inhibitor. Statins inhibit the action of the enzyme HMG-CoA reductase, blocking the manufacture of cholesterol in the body, mainly in the liver.

Sterols: Phytosterols; compounds that are very similar to cholesterol but occur in plants rather than in animals. Their cholesterol-lowering effects were first reported in the 1950s.

Stroke: Also call "brain attack," a stroke is a loss of blood flow to a part of the brain causing death of brain tissue and loss of one or more functions, including weakness, paralysis, loss of sensation or coordination, or the ability to speak or see. Stroke can be due to a blockage in a blood vessel, a blood clot, or bleeding into part of the brain.

T

Total cholesterol: The measure of LDL cholesterol, HDL cholesterol, and other lipid components.

Transient ischemic attack (TIA): Transient (or temporary) neurologic symptoms.

Triglycerides: Lipids that are stored in fat cells and used as a source of energy. Triglycerides may be either made by the liver or ingested through the diet. Elevated blood plasma levels of these lipids are positively correlated with coronary heart disease risk and are thought to contribute to atherosclerosis.

V

Very-low-density lipoprotein (VLDL): Lipoprotein made in the liver that contains mostly triglycerides and some cholesterol.